ONE

Respiratory System

One Stop Doc

Titles in the series include:

Cardiovascular System – Jonathan Aron
Editorial Advisor – Jeremy Ward

Cell and Molecular Biology – Desikan Rangarajan and David Shaw
Editorial Advisor – Barbara Moreland

Endocrine and Reproductive Systems – Caroline Jewels and Alexandra Tillett
Editorial Advisor – Stuart Milligan

Gastrointestinal System – Miruna Canagaratnam
Editorial Advisor – Richard Naftalin

Musculoskeletal System – Wayne Lam, Bassel Zebian and Rishi Aggarwal
Editorial Advisor – Alistair Hunter

Nervous System – Elliott Smock
Editorial Advisor – Clive Coen

Metabolism and Nutrition – Miruna Canagaratnam and David Shaw
Editorial Advisors – Barbara Moreland and Richard Naftalin

Renal and Urinary System and Electrolyte Balance – Panos Stamoulos and Spyros Bakalis
Editorial Advisors – Alistair Hunter and Richard Naftalin

ONE STOP DOC

Respiratory System

Jo Dartnell BSc(Hons)
Fifth year medical student, Guy's, King's and
St Thomas' Medical School, London, UK

Michelle Ramsay BSc(Hons)
Fifth year medical student, Guy's, King's and
St Thomas' Medical School, London, UK

Editorial Advisor: John Rees MD FRCP
Consultant Physician, Senior Lecturer in Medicine, Guy's, King's and
St Thomas' Medical School, London, UK

Series Editor: Elliott Smock BSc(Hons)
Fifth year medical student, Guy's, King's and
St Thomas' Medical School, London, UK

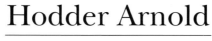

Hodder Arnold

A MEMBER OF THE HODDER HEADLINE GROUP

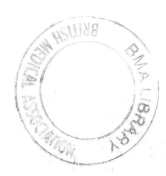

First published in Great Britain in 2005 by
Hodder Education, a member of the Hodder Headline Group,
338 Euston Road, London NW1 3BH

http://www.hoddereducation.co.uk

Distributed in the United States of America by
Oxford University Press Inc.,
198 Madison Avenue, New York, NY10016
Oxford is a registered trademark of Oxford University Press

Whilst the advice and information in this book are believed to be true and
accurate at the date of going to press, neither the authors nor the publisher
can accept any legal responsibility or liability for any errors or omissions
that may be made. In particular, (but without limiting the generality of the
preceding disclaimer) every effort has been made to check drug dosages;
however it is still possible that errors have been missed. Furthermore,
dosage schedules are constantly being revised and new side-effects
recognized. For these reasons the reader is strongly urged to consult the
drug companies' printed instructions before administering any of the drugs
recommended in this book.

British Library Cataloguing in Publication Data
A catalogue record for this book is available from the British Library

Library of Congress Cataloging-in-Publication Data
A catalog record for this book is available from the Library of Congress

ISBN-10: 0 340 88504 1
ISBN-13: 978 0 340 88504 8

1 2 3 4 5 6 7 8 9 10

Commissioning Editor: Georgina Bentliff
Project Editor: Heather Smith
Production Controller: Jane Lawrence
Cover Design: Amina Dudhia
Illustrations: Cactus Design
Index: Indexing Specialists (UK) Ltd

Typeset in 10/12pt Adobe Garamond/Akzidenz GroteskBE by Servis Filmsetting Ltd, Manchester
Printed and bound in Spain

Hodder Headline's policy is to use papers that are natural, renewable and recyclable
products and made from wood grown in sustainable forests. The logging and manufacturing processes are
expected to conform to the environmental regulations of the country of origin.

What do you think about this book? Or any other Hodder Arnold title?
Please visit our website at **www.hoddereducation.co.uk**

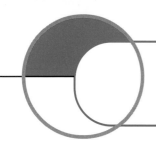

CONTENTS

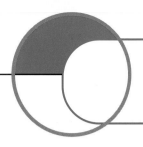

PREFACE

From the Series Editor, Elliott Smock

Are you ready to face your looming exams? If you have done loads of work, then congratulations; we hope this opportunity to practice SAQs, EMQs, MCQs and Problem-based Questions on every part of the core curriculum will help you consolidate what you've learnt and improve your exam technique. If you don't feel ready, don't panic – the One Stop Doc series has all the answers you need to catch up and pass.

There are only a limited number of questions an examiner can throw at a beleaguered student and this text can turn that to your advantage. By getting straight into the heart of the core questions that come up year after year and by giving you the model answers you need this book will arm you with the knowledge to succeed in your exams. Broken down into logical sections, you can learn all the important facts you need to pass without having to wade through tons of different textbooks when you simply don't have the time. All questions presented here are 'core'; those of the highest importance have been highlighted to allow even sharper focus if time for revision is running out. In addition, to allow you to organize your revision efficiently, questions have been grouped by topic, with answers supported by detailed integrated explanations.

On behalf of all the One Stop Doc authors I wish you the very best of luck in your exams and hope these books serve you well!

From the Authors, Jo Dartnell and Michelle Ramsay

The respiratory system will form an enormous part of your medical training. It is essential to get to grips with the basics of anatomy, physiology, pharmacology and disease processes early on. This book will hopefully act as a guide through these sometimes difficult concepts!

We've divided the book into 4 simplistic sections which cover topics often examined but not well covered in other textbooks. Section 1 covers the upper respiratory tract which is often forgotten, but very important. Section 2 is the lower respiratory tract and the mechanics of breathing. Section 3 contains some of the more complex physiological material. As more courses are becoming clinical from an early stage, section 4 covers in depth the basis of common conditions you should know.

We would like to thank Dr John Rees for his time and help in reviewing our work on many occasions. Also we are grateful to Elliott Smock, for the opportunity to write a textbook and for trusting us to do it! Finally thanks to our families and friends who never believed that we'd actually pull this off!

We wish you the best of luck in your exams and hope you find this book helpful!

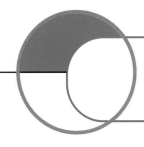

ABBREVIATIONS

ACh	acetylcholine
ADP	adenosine diphosphate
APUD	amine precursor uptake and decarboxylation
ATP	adenosine triphosphate
BALT	bronchus-associated lymphoid tissue
BCG	Bacille Calmette-Guerín
BP	blood pressure
cAMP	cyclic adenosine monophosphate
CF	cystic fibrosis
CFTR	cystic fibrosis transmembrane conductance regulator
COPD	chronic obstructive pulmonary disease
CPAP	continuous positive airway pressure
CSF	cerebrospinal fluid
CT	computed tomography
2,3-DPG	2,3-diphosphoglycerate
EEG	electroencephalogram
EGF	epidermal growth factor
Exp.RV	expiratory reserve volume
FBC	full blood count
FEV_1	forced expiratory volume in 1 s
FGF	fibroblast growth factor
Fn.RV	functional residual volume
FVC	forced vital capacity
GP	general practitioner
GI	gastrointestinal
Hb	haemoglobin
HbA	adult haemoglobin
HbF	fetal haemoglobin
IgA	immunoglobulin A
IL	interleukin
Insp.RV	inspiratory reserve volume
ITP	immunoreactive trypsin test
LFT	liver function test
MRI	magnetic resonance imaging
NSAID	non-steroidal anti-inflammatory drug
OSA	obstructive sleep apnoea
$Paco_2$	arterial partial pressure of carbon dioxide
PEFR	peak expiratory flow rate
Po_2	partial pressure of oxygen
$\dot{Q}$	perfusion
RBC	red blood cell
RV	residual volume
TB	tuberculosis
Th_2	T helper type 2 lymphocytes
TLC	total lung capacity
TV	tidal volume
$\dot{V}_A$	minute alvolar ventilation
$\dot{V}_E$	minute ventilation
VC	vital capacity

UPPER RESPIRATORY TRACT

UPPER RESPIRATORY TRACT

1. Functions of the upper respiratory tract include

a. Speech

b. Smell

c. Warming incoming air

d. Dehumidifying incoming air

e. Swallowing

2. Concerning the nasal cavity

a. It is bounded inferiorly by the hard palate

b. The maxillary sinuses lie superiorly

c. It is lined with respiratory epithelium

d. Its main function is to warm and dry the incoming air

e. It is prone to infection

3. Concerning the nasal conchae

a. They are made of cartilage

b. The maxillary sinuses open into the middle meatus

c. The nasolacrimal duct drains into the inferior meatus

d. The ethmoidal sinuses open into the middle and inferior meatuses

e. The conchae are highly vascular

4. Match 1–5 on the coronal section of the skull with one of the options below

Options

A. Sphenoidal sinus

B. Frontal sinus

C. Ethmoidal sinus

D. Maxillary sinus

E. Superior meatus

F. Middle meatus

G. Inferior meatus

H. Sphenoethmoidal recess

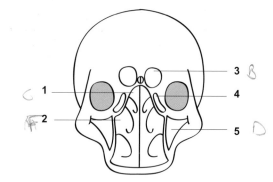

EXPLANATION: FUNCTIONS OF THE UPPER RESPIRATORY TRACT

The upper respiratory tract extends from the **nose/mouth** down to the lower border of the **cricoid** cartilage. Therefore **speech** and **smell** are included in its functions. Gas exchange is more efficient in warmer and wetter air, so air is **warmed** and **moistened** as it passes through the nasal cavity and mouth.

The figure below shows how the nasal cavity is bordered **inferiorly** by the **hard palate**, **laterally** by the **maxillary** and **ethmoidal sinuses** and **superiorly** by the **frontal** and **sphenoidal sinuses**. It contains three **conchae/turbinates** which increase the surface area through which the air must pass to be warmed and moistened. The cavity is lined with **respiratory epithelium** which contains mucous glands and is highly vascular. The sinuses are prone to infection (sinusitis).

The conchae are made of thin sheets of bone and create three meatuses: inferior, middle and superior. The inferior meatus contains the opening for the nasolacrimal duct (which is why when you cry your nose runs), the middle meatus contains openings to the ethmoidal and maxillary sinuses and the frontal nasal ducts and the superior meatus has another opening for the ethmoidal sinuses. Like the rest of the cavity the conchae are lined with respiratory epithelium containing many blood vessels.

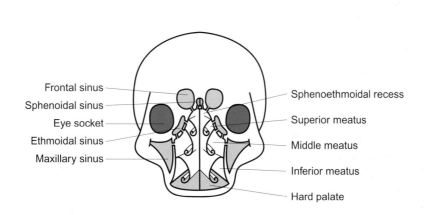

5. Concerning the pharynx

a. It receives blood from the external carotid artery
b. Pharyngeal venous blood drains straight into the superior vena cava
c. It is drained by deep cervical lymph nodes
d. It is innervated by the maxillary nerve
e. It is only supplied by motor neurons

6. The nasopharynx

a. Begins at the entrance to the nose
b. Ensures smooth flow of air
c. Has columnar ciliated epithelium
d. Is connected to the auditory canal
e. Can be occluded by the soft palate

7. Concerning the oropharynx and laryngopharynx

a. The laryngopharynx joins to the oropharynx
b. The oropharynx continues down the oesophagus
c. The laryngopharynx opens into the oesophagus
d. They include the epiglottis
e. The epiglottis occludes the oesophagus during breathing

EXPLANATION: THE PHARYNX AND LARYNX (i)

The **external carotid artery** supplies the pharynx through several smaller tributaries. The **internal jugular vein** receives the venous blood before draining into the superior vena cava. Lymphatic drainage is into the **deep cervical lymph nodes**. Sensory branches of the maxillary nerve (Vth cranial nerve) supply the nasopharynx, but the main innervation of the pharynx is by the **pharyngeal plexus**. This comprises motor and sensory branches of the glossopharyngeal (IXth) and vagus (Xth) nerves.

The first part of the pharynx, the **nasopharynx**, begins posteriorly at its attachment to the sphenoid bone at the base of the skull, and anteriorly where the nasal septum ends at a point known as the posterior choana. From there it takes a 90° turn downwards and so increases air turbulence. This helps further impaction and removal of particles. This is also the transition point from columnar ciliated epithelium to **squamous cells**. The eustachian tube exits in the nasopharynx, which explains the link between concurrent upper respiratory tract and ear infections. The soft palate rises during swallowing to occlude the nasal cavity entrance. The epiglottis occludes the lower respiratory tract during swallowing. This prevents foreign objects being aspirated up into the nasal cavity.

The nasopharynx ends at the lower border of the soft palate and the **oropharynx** starts. The oropharynx continues into the **laryngopharynx**. One of the functions of the pharynx, as well as allowing the passage of air into the trachea, is to carry food and drink to the oesophagus. It ends at the start of the oesophagus, at the level of the cricoid cartilage, and the larynx, after the epiglottis.

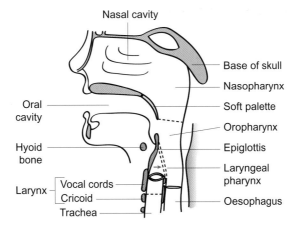

Answers

5. T F T F F
6. F F F T T
7. T F T T F

8. The oropharynx and laryngopharynx epithelium

 a. Is covered by respiratory epithelium
 b. Is keratinized
 c. Consists of squamous cells
 d. It is one cell thick
 e. Contains many goblet cells

9. The larynx has an important role in

 a. Regulation of air flow
 b. Phonation
 c. Occluding the trachea
 d. Stimulation of the cough reflex
 e. The Valsalva manoevure

10. Consider the larynx

 a. The superior and inferior laryngeal arteries supply the larynx
 b. Branches of the vagus nerve supply the larynx
 c. The mucosa above the vocal cords is innervated by the internal superior laryngeal nerve
 d. The intrinsic muscles are supplied by the recurrent laryngeal nerve
 e. The cricothyroid muscle is supplied by the external superior laryngeal nerve

11. Consider the larynx epithelium

 a. It is covered by respiratory epithelium
 b. It is made up of non-keratinized squamous cells above the vocal cords
 c. Keratinized squamous cells line the vocal cords
 d. It helps remove mucus by ciliary action
 e. It joins up with the tracheal epithelium with a definite border

EXPLANATION: THE PHARYNX AND LARYNX (ii)

Non-keratinized epithelium lines the oropharynx and laryngopharynx as it is part of the alimentary tract as well as respiratory tissue. There are multiple layers of this epithelium which are kept moist by saliva from the many salivary glands.

Air passes through the larynx to reach the lungs, but the vocal cords must be open for this to occur, therefore it acts to **regulate air flow**. Someone who has had their larynx removed is unable to produce normal speech. The larynx is vital in protecting the lower respiratory tract during swallowing and vomiting. The vocal cords close, thereby causing the epiglottis to move backwards and obscure the entrance. Mucus and foreign particles reaching the larynx stimulate the **cough reflex**. This is important in allowing clearance of mucus from the lungs. The **Valsalva manoeuvre** is where the diaphragm is fixed and the larynx closes to allow intra-abdominal pressure to rise, for example during defecation.

The blood supply for the larynx comes from the **superior** and **inferior laryngeal arteries**. Branches of the **vagus** (Xth cranial) nerve and the **recurrent** and **superior laryngeal nerves** provide the innervation. The **internal superior laryngeal** nerve supplies the mucosa **above** the vocal cords. The area **below** is supplied by the **recurrent laryngeal nerve**, which also supplies the internal intrinsic muscles (interarytenoid, thyroarytenoid, aryepiglottic, cricoarytenoid, thyroepiglottic). This nerve can be damaged during thyroid surgery so altering the movement of the vocal cord on that side. The external superior laryngeal nerve supplies the external muscle (cricothyroid).

The area of the larynx above and including the vestibular and vocal folds is lined by **non-keratinized squamous** epithelium. There are no cilia here, so removal of mucus relies on musculoskeletal means – i.e. coughing, see page 13. Below the cords, **respiratory epithelium** restarts which is continuous with the trachea.

Answers
8. F F F F F
9. T T T T T
10. T T T T T
11. F T F F F

12. Complete the following paragraph with one of the options from the list below. Each option can be used once, more than once or not at all

Options

A. Epiglottic cartilage
C. Thyroid cartilage
E. Laryngeal cartilage
G. Medially

B. Hyoid bone
D. Cricoid cartilage
F. Arytenoid cartilage
H. Laterally

The larynx is mainly surrounded by the **1**. This is made of hyaline cartilage, whilst the **2** is elastic cartilage. On the posterior rim of the **3** sit the two **4**, to which the vocal cords attach posteriorly. These rotate **5** to open the trachea and **6** to shut it. An emergency tracheostomy must be inserted through the ligament connecting the **7** and **8** to avoid damage to the vocal cords.

13. The diagram below is a longitudinal section through the larynx. Label it using the following options

Options

A. The true (vocal) fold
C. The aryepiglottic fold
E. The thyroid cartilage

B. The false (vestibular) fold
D. The cricoid cartilage,
F. The arytenoid cartilage

Anterior ←

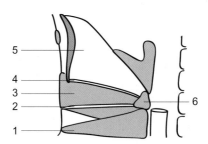

14. What is the name of the ligament mainly responsible for altering the tension on the vocal cords?

EXPLANATION: THE LARYNX

The mucous membrane connecting the cartilage box surrounding the larynx is strengthened with collagen and forms three pairs of folds: the **aryepiglottic** (superior), **vestibular/false** (middle) and **vocal/true** (inferior) folds. These are an important defence mechanism for the larynx.

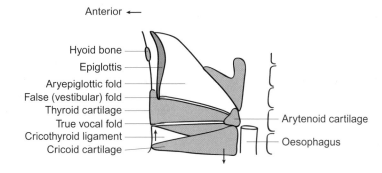

The larynx is surrounded by the **thyroid cartilage**, which is inferiorly attached to the **cricoid cartilage** by the **cricothyroid ligament (14)**. It is this that contracts and pulls the anterior part of the cricoid upwards. The posterior end rocks backwards taking the arytenoid cartilage with it. Therefore the tension on the vocal cords increases. This is shown by the arrows on the above diagram **(14)**.

The figure below shows the view that anaesthetists look for when intubating a patient to ensure the tube passes into the trachea and not down the oesophagus. You can see that when the arytenoid cartilages rotate laterally the cords open, and rotation medially (purple arrows) causes them to close thus protecting the airway.

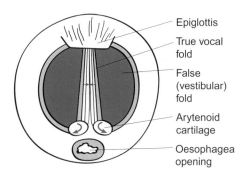

Answers

12. 1 – C, 2 – A, 3 – D, 4 – F, 5 – H, 6 – G, 7 – C/D, 8 – C/D
13. 1 – D, 2 – A, 3 – E, 4 – B, 5 – C, 6 – F
14. See explanation

15. Snoring

    a. Is due to increased pharyngeal skeletal muscle tone
    b. Occurs on inspiration and expiration
    c. Obesity is a predisposing factor
    d. Is more common in females
    e. Causes $PaCO_2$ to rise

16. Obstructive sleep apnoea

    a. Is very rare
    b. Is more common in males
    c. Is associated with hypertension
    d. Causes the patient to wake up
    e. Causes pulmonary hypertension

17. Concerning treatment of sleep-disordered breathing

    a. First-line treatment is surgery
    b. All patients should try to avoid sleeping on their backs
    c. O_2 cures snoring and obstructive sleep apnoea
    d. Patients should be prescribed sleeping tablets
    e. Nocturnal continuous positive airway pressure is a last resort

---

CPAP, continuous positive airway pressure; EEG, electroencephalogram; OSA, obstructive sleep apnoea; $PaCO_2$, arterial partial pressure of carbon dioxide

EXPLANATION: SLEEP-DISORDERED BREATHING

General skeletal muscle tone decreases during sleep, leading to the pharyngeal walls and soft palate collapsing on themselves, so preventing normal air flow. The classical snoring noise is heard during inspiration, but can be heard on expiration. Obese patients and those who sleep on their backs snore the most. During normal sleep $PaCO_2$ rises slightly. In snorers, $PaCO_2$ increases abnormally which adds to the problem as it causes the patient to inhale even more deeply.

OSA is common and affects approximately 1 in 25 people. It is normal to have a few episodes of OSA each night. Risk factors include obesity, increasing age, alcohol consumption, male sex, hypothyroidism and hypertension. Rising blood pressure is also noted during the apnoeic episode, peaking when respiration stops. The patient is at increased risk of stroke during this period especially if they are already hypertensive. OSA doesn't actually wake the patient, but causes changes on the EEG – an **EEG arousal**. This leads to the patient spontaneously breathing normally often after changing position. Severe OSA can lead to pulmonary hypertension due to hypoxia causing pulmonary vasoconstriction.

First-line treatment should only be surgical if there is an anatomical abnormality; other methods of management should be considered first in other cases. Many patients who snore can be helped by preventing them from sleeping on their backs, to stop the tongue falling backwards. O_2 prevents hypoxia but does not cure the problem. Although these patients sleep badly, sleeping tablets should not be prescribed as they may prevent arousal from an apnoeic period, they can depress respiration and they make sleep apnoea worse. Nocturnal CPAP helps many patients by keeping the pharynx inflated. It is usually administered via a nasal or full face mask. This is not an easy treatment option and compliance by the patient is often poor.

Answers

15. F T T F T
16. F T T F T
17. F T F F F

18. Consider the cough reflex

a. It is stimulated by increased bronchiolar mucus
b. Irritant receptors are found throughout the respiratory tract
c. Messages are sent to the respiratory centre via the vagus nerve
d. The phrenic nerve is involved in the reflex
e. The larynx is just responsible for making the coughing sound

19. Regarding the sneeze reflex

a. It is stimulated by receptors in the nasal cavity
b. The respiratory centre is stimulated by the vagus to initiate the sneeze
c. The hindbrain needs to be intact for the reflex
d. The soft palate rises on the forced expiration
e. Nasal mucus is reflexly increased

EXPLANATION: REFLEXES

When the **irritant receptors**, which are found throughout the respiratory tract, are stimulated in the larynx, trachea and main bronchi, the **cough reflex** is initiated. Stimulation lower down the tract causes hyperpnoea (breathing too fast). The receptors send messages via the **vagi** to the respiratory centre which sends the message to the nerves innervating the muscles of respiration, i.e. **phrenic** (diaphragm), **intercostal** (intercostal muscles) and **lumbar nerves** (abdominal muscles). Therefore all nerve roots from C3 to L3 are involved! The vagus also sends a message to the larynx causing the glottis to **close**, which increases the intrathoracic pressure. As the larynx opens, the irritant is forced out of the respiratory tract through the nose or mouth.

If irritant receptors in the nasal cavity are stimulated, they send messages via the **trigeminal** (Vth) nerve to the general sensory nucleus in the hindbrain. They are then directed on to the respiratory centre, which sends information to the muscles of respiration. Following a forced expiration the tongue (via the hypoglossal (XIIth) nerve) and soft palate (via the Xth nerve) are elevated, so occluding the pharynx and forcing the air and irritant out from the pharynx. In contrast to the cough the glottis stays **open**. We have all experienced the increase in nasal mucus I'm sure! This is via the parasympathetic efferents of the facial (VIIth) nerve to the glands in the nasal mucous membrane.

Answers
18. F T T T F
19. T F T T T

LOWER RESPIRATORY TRACT

1. During development

- **a.** The lungs originate from ectoderm in the developing fetus
- **b.** The lungs start to develop before the heart
- **c.** The trachea and main bronchi develop first followed by smaller bronchi
- **d.** The bronchial cartilage and smooth muscle develop from the mesoderm
- **e.** Respiratory bronchioles develop by week 24

2. Lung development

- **a.** Type I alveolar pneumocytes are important to enable future gas exchange in the lung
- **b.** Type II alveolar pneumocytes are found in the terminal bronchiole sacs
- **c.** Surfactant is produced by type II pneumocytes following the infant's first breath
- **d.** Glucocorticoids may be given to the mother to stimulate fetal surfactant production
- **e.** Neonatal respiratory distress syndrome only occurs in infants born before 24 weeks

3. Regarding lung development

- **a.** Alveoli form from week 32 onwards
- **b.** Mature alveoli are present from birth
- **c.** Infants are born with a number of alveoli fixed for life
- **d.** Fetal breathing can be observed inside the uterus
- **e.** Lung development is dependent on the level of amniotic fluid in the uterus

4. At birth

- **a.** The lungs are 50 per cent full of fluid
- **b.** Surfactant enables air to fill and expand the alveoli
- **c.** Arterial O_2 decreases
- **d.** The vascular resistance of the pulmonary circulation is reduced below that of the systemic circulation
- **e.** Blood flows through the foramen ovale to reach the lungs

EGF, epidermal growth factor; FGF, fibroblast growth factor

EXPLANATION: EMBRYOLOGICAL ORIGINS OF THE LOWER RESPIRATORY SYSTEM

The respiratory system originates from both the **endoderm** and the **mesoderm.** The endoderm develops into the epithelium and glands of the larynx, trachea and the lungs. The mesoderm forms the tracheal cartilage, smooth muscle, lung parenchyma and connective tissue. The lungs develop by a process called branching morphogenesis which relies on signalling molecules such as FGF and EGF for accurate positioning.

Initial development starts in week four with the formation of a **laryngotracheal tube** (known as the **embryonic phase**). By the end of week four, the laryngotracheal tube bifurcates into two **bronchial buds** which form the primitive right and left main bronchi. The second stage of development is the **pseudoglandular phase** which lasts from weeks 5 to 17. During this time multiple smaller **bronchi** form.

From week 16 to week 25 (the **canalicular phase**), the bronchioles form and divide into smaller **alveolar ducts** and **terminal sacs**. **Type I pneumocytes** form a squamous epithelium that lines the terminal sacs and combines with capillaries to form a future gas exchange surface. A few **type II pneumocytes** are also present in the terminal sacs. These cells secrete small amounts of surfactant from week 20, however there is insufficient to support life until after 28 weeks of gestation. Insufficient surfactant leads to respiratory distress syndrome in the neonate which has a significant mortality as air cannot enter the alveoli and so oxygenation does not occur. If a pre-term delivery is expected, glucocorticoids can be given to the mother antenatally to stimulate fetal surfactant production.

The **saccular phase** occurs from week 24 until birth. During this time the number of terminal sacs increases rapidly and immature alveoli begin to form from week 32.

The **alveolar phase** occurs from the late fetal period until childhood. During this time the alveoli mature and increase in size and number, causing the lungs to enlarge.

While in the uterus the fetus begins breathing movements, inhaling the surrounding amniotic fluid which stimulates lung growth. At birth, air fills the lungs and enters the alveoli for gas exchange if there is sufficient surfactant to keep them open. As the infant takes its first breath, the arterial O_2 increases, which reduces the pulmonary vascular resistance below that of the systemic circulation. This enables more blood to flow into the lungs causing the pressure gradient across the foramen ovale in the heart to reverse. This results in closure of the foramen ovale.

Answers

1. F F T T T
2. T T F T F
3. T F F T T
4. T T F T F

5. Functions of the lower respiratory tract include

    a. O_2 exchange between the blood and air
    b. Regulating the acid–base balance in the body
    c. Angiotensin I conversion to angiotensin II
    d. Activation of neurotransmitters such as serotonin, noradrenaline and ACh
    e. Good defence against pathogens

6. Other functions include

    a. Temperature regulation
    b. Loss of water
    c. Matching respiration to behaviour
    d. Metabolism of drugs
    e. Filtration of microemboli from systemic veins

ACh, acetylcholine

EXPLANATION: FUNCTIONS OF THE LOWER RESPIRATORY TRACT

O_2 and CO_2 are exchanged between the blood and atmosphere. There is little point of one without the other. The respiratory system is of vital importance in regulating the acid–base balance of the body. This is done by monitoring the levels of CO_2 and **pH** in the body. Neurotransmitters and drugs such as propranolol and chlorpromazine are removed or **deactivated** in the lung. The lungs produce mucus as a **partial barrier** to infection and foreign material. However the vast surface area of the lungs and the fact they are open to the environment means that they are very susceptible to infection and injury from foreign materials.

By altering ventilation, body temperature can be regulated to an extent, i.e. when we are hot we breathe more. As the surface of the lungs needs to be wet for effective gas exchange, loss of water in expired air is inevitable. Mucus is secreted to try and prevent this, but when calculating a patient's fluid balance, water loss through respiration must be taken into consideration. **Ventilation is increased** to match the body's metabolism to ensure enough O_2 is present. Drugs such as amphetamine and imipramine are taken up and metabolized by the lung. The lungs can filter **microemboli**, however larger emboli block blood vessels and lead to pulmonary embolism.

Answers
5. T T T F F
6. T F T T T

7. Regarding the surface anatomy of the lower respiratory tract

    a. The trachea divides at the level of the angle of Louis
    b. The trachea divides at the level of the second rib
    c. The angle of Louis is in the same horizontal plane as the T2 vertebra
    d. The clavicles are above the apices of the lungs
    e. On full expiration, the lungs extend down to the tenth rib
    f. The visceral pleura extend down below the tenth rib

8. Match the ribs in the list with their respective lung lobes, using the options given

Options

    1. Anterior right third rib
    2. Posterior left third rib
    3. Posterior left third rib
    4. Anterior right fifth rib
    5. Posterior right seventh rib

    A. Right upper lobe
    B. Right middle lobe
    C. Right lower lobe
    D. Left upper lobe
    E. Left middle lobe
    F. Left lower lobe

EXPLANATION: SURFACE ANATOMY (i)

The angle of Louis is where the **manubrium** meets the body of the **sternum**. This is the surface marking for the bifurcation of the trachea and also the second rib. Horizontally it is in the same plane as the fourth thoracic vertebra (**T4**). The apex of each lung rises above the medial third of the clavicle. The lungs normally end around the **eighth rib** but on full expiration can extend down towards the tenth rib but not quite that far. The **visceral pleura** cover the surface of the lung, whereas the **parietal pleura** cover the internal thoracic cavity and extend down below the tenth rib. From the diagram below of a lateral view of the right lung, see how the sixth rib is crossed by the inferior lung border in the mid-clavicular line and the eighth rib in the mid-axillary line. The lowest border is posteriorly at the tenth rib.

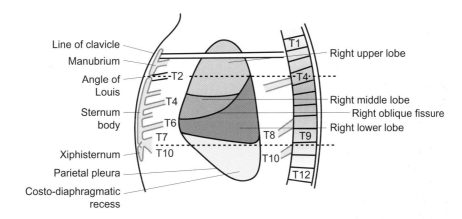

The fissures on the lungs are shown on the X-ray below. The oblique fissures are not seen on the postero-anterior chest X-ray.

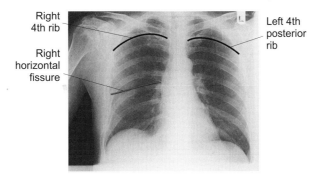

From Aron, A., *One Stop Doc Cardiovascular System*, Arnold 2004.

Answers
7. T T F F F F
8. 1 – A, 2 – D, 3 – F, 4 – B, 5 – C

9. On both the diagrams below label

a. The visceral pleura
b. The parietal pleura
c. The costodiaphragmatic recess
d. The two oblique fissures and single horizontal fissure
e. Draw the tracheal bifurcation on the anterior view
f. On a male patient what is the surface marking for the middle lobe?

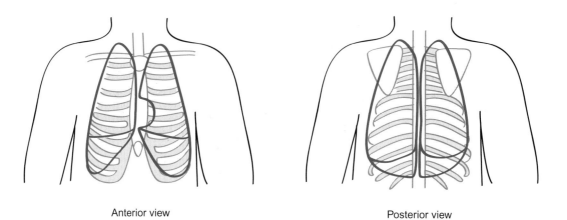

Anterior view

Posterior view

10. On the X-ray below

a. Label the fourth rib
b. Draw the positions of the fissures in the right and left lungs

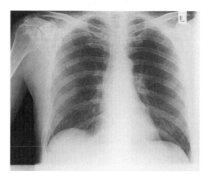

From Aron, A., *One Stop Doc Cardiovascular System*, Arnold 2004.

EXPLANATION: SURFACE ANATOMY (ii)

The part of the pleural cavity not occupied by the lung is called the **costodiaphragmatic recess**. Passing a needle through the eighth or ninth intercostal space, will avoid the lungs as long as the patient doesn't breathe in fully. Consequently it is the choice site for a liver biopsy.

On a non-obese male patient the **horizontal fissure** is in line with the right nipple. Placing the palm of your hand below it covers the middle lobe. You can therefore work out where the lower lobes are.

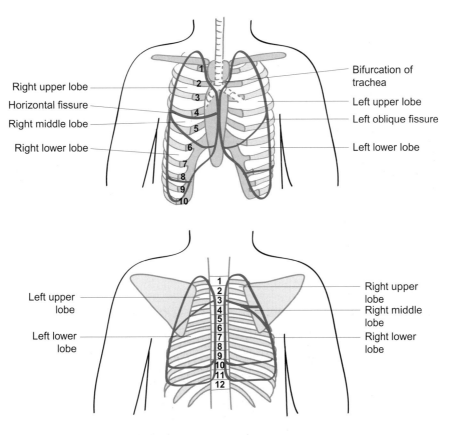

Answers

9. See figure
10. Trick question! The oblique fissures are not seen on a normal postero–anterior chest X-ray, but need a lateral view (see diagram on page 21)

11. Regarding the basic anatomy of the lower respiratory tract

a. The upper respiratory tract ends at the bifurcation of the trachea
b. Bony horseshoe-shaped rings surround the anterior and lateral aspects of the trachea
c. The bifurcation of the trachea is known as the carina
d. The right main bronchus is at greater risk than the left of becoming obstructed by an inhaled foreign object
e. Bronchi have walls of cartilage and smooth muscle

12. The respiratory epithelium contains

a. Goblet cells
b. Squamous cells
c. Ciliated columnar cells
d. Keratinocytes
e. Basal cells

EXPLANATION: ANATOMY AND HISTOLOGY OF THE LOWER RESPIRATORY TRACT

The upper respiratory tract contains the nose, pharynx and larynx and ends at the lower border of the cricoid cartilage. **Cartilaginous** horseshoe-shaped rings support the anterior and lateral trachea. The point at which the trachea bifurcates is the **carina**. The left main bronchus branches off the trachea at a more oblique angle than the right, which is more in line with the trachea. Inhaled foreign objects are therefore more likely to 'fall' straight down and block the **right** side as it is more vertical than the left. The smooth muscle in the bronchi walls is on the internal surface of the cartilaginous rings and as the rings fade out, more smooth muscle is found. It is this smooth muscle that is affected in **asthma** and acted upon by **bronchdilators**.

The respiratory epithelium changes slightly as it progresses through the respiratory tract, although its main components remain the same, see below. The upper third of the nasal cavity is **olfactory epithelium** and will not be covered. Excluding the oropharynx and laryngopharynx, the lower two-thirds of the nasal cavity up to the terminal bronchioles is lined with pseudostratified, **ciliated columnar epithelium**. Goblet (mucus-secreting) **cells** are scattered through this and have microvilli on their surface. These cells secrete mucus which sticks to inhaled dust particles, etc. It is then propelled upwards by the cilia to the larynx where it initiates the cough reflex and the mucus is coughed up and swallowed. This is known as the **mucociliary escalator**. However, these are normally not present in terminal bronchioles and here the cells are more cuboidal than columnar. Immature **basal cells** are found next to the **basement membrane** and divide to replace any other cells that die.

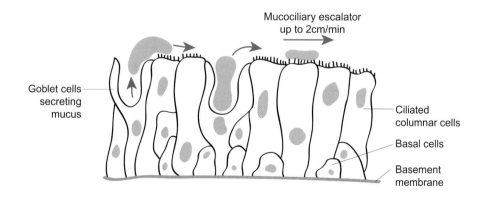

Answers
11. F F T T T
12. T F T F T

13. Label the layers in the figure below from the list below

Options

A. Mucosa
B. Submucosa
C. Epithelium
D. Lamina propria
E. Basement membrane
F. Cartilage

14. Consider the figure below

a. Given that this is a section from the trachea. List two ways in which the bronchus, bronchiole and terminal bronchiole are different
b. The alveoli have different epithelium. How is it different and why?
c. What is the function of the cells making up the epithelium?

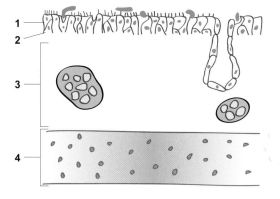

EXPLANATION: LOWER RESPIRATORY TRACT EPITHELIUM

The gap in the horseshoe cartilage of the trachea is joined by a dense fibrocartilaginous ligament which allows constriction but prevents dilation of the trachea.

The **bronchus** walls also have respiratory epithelium but here it contains smooth muscle as well making contraction possible. The cartilage around them is incomplete compared with the horseshoe-shape in the trachea. This allows space for contraction of the smooth muscle.

The **bronchiole** walls do not contain cartilage or mucous glands, but have the smooth muscle. The epithelial cells are more cuboidal than columnar **(14a)**.

The **terminal bronchioles** are similar to the bronchioles but the cells are further flattened and can allow some gas exchange **(14a)**.

Alveoli walls are made of respiratory cells known as pneumocytes of which there are two types I and II **(14b)**. These lie flat against the basement membrane making a very thin blood–air interface, very suitable for their function of gas exchange. Type I cells are structural while type II produce surfactant **(14c)** – see page 41. There is no smooth muscle in the wall so alveoli are non-contractile.

Answers
13. 1 – C, 2 – E, 3 – B, 4 – F
14. See explanation

15. Below is a drawing of a cross-section through the thorax at the level of T10. Match up 1–13 with one of the list below. Each may be used once, more than once or not at all

Options

A. Trachea
B. Descending aorta
C. Oesophagus
D. Superior vena cava
E. Inferior vena cava
F. Left phrenic nerve
G. Right phrenic nerve
H. Central tendon
I. Medial arcuate ligament

J. Right vagus nerve
K. Left vagus nerve
L. Pericardial sac
M. Visceral pleura
N. Parietal pleura
O. Diaphragmatic pleura
P. Xiphisternum
Q. Costodiaphragmatic recess
R. Body of sternum

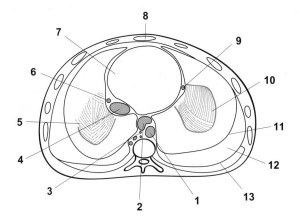

EXPLANATION: CROSS-SECTIONAL ANATOMY

Cross-sectional imaging is becoming a popular way of testing anatomy in preparation for interpreting CT scans. When looking at an image, imagine the patient lying flat on their back with their feet coming out of the page and their head going away from you. This way, confusing right and left will never be a problem. This is a very different way of learning anatomy and just takes practice!

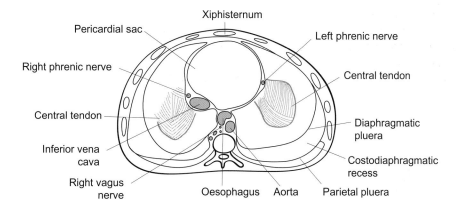

CT uses X-rays to produce a picture which differentiates the structures by their densities. Bone is high density whilst air and fat are low density structures. By injecting a contrast agent intravenously, anything containing blood is shown up. CT is useful for imaging lymph nodes, pulmonary embolism and cancers. Staging of tumours is also very dependent on CT scanning. The lung parenchyma can be seen in more detail and CT is very useful to evaluate pulmonary fibrosis, bronchiectasis and the extent and distribution of emphysema.

Answers

15. 1 – B, 2 – C, 3 – J, 4 – E, 5 – H, 6 – G, 7 – L, 8 – P, 9 – F, 10 – H, 11 – O, 12 – Q, 13 – N

16. Consider the rib cage

    a. Only ribs one to ten are connected to the sternum
    b. Ribs nine and ten articulate with the xiphisternum
    c. The manubriosternal joint is also known as the angle of Louis
    d. The first two ribs are those most likely to fracture
    e. A person with arm parasthesiae or vascular problems may have a cervical rib

17. Consider the thoracic cage

    a. The manubrium is divided into three parts
    b. Only the first seven ribs articulate directly with the sternum along its lateral borders
    c. The weakest part of the rib is at its angle
    d. The upper border of each rib has a groove running along it in which the neurovascular bundle can be found
    e. The external intercostal muscles contain fibres which run downwards and anteriorly

18. **Below is a diagram of a typical rib. Label 1–9 from the list. Each answer may be used once, more than once or not at all**

Options

    A. Attaches to the corresponding vertebra
    B. Attaches to the costal cartilage
    C. Attaches to the clavicle
    D. Attaches to the transverse process of the vertebra
    E. Attaches to the vertebra above
    F. Head
    G. Neck
    H. Body
    I. Shaft
    J. Tubercle
    K. Costal groove
    L. Costal margin
    M. Pleural groove

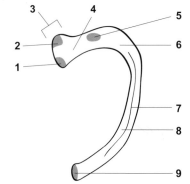

EXPLANATION: THE CHEST WALL

The chest wall comprises the **sternum, ribs, intercostal muscles** and the **thoracic vertebral column**. Ribs one to ten are connected to the sternum. Ribs 11 and 12 do not attach are termed 'free-floating' ribs. The sternum is made up of the **manubrium** (attaches the clavicle, rib one and half of rib two), the **body** (attaches ribs three to ten) and the cartilaginous **xiphisternum**. The manubrio-sternal joint is also known as **the angle of Louis**. The first two ribs are protected under the clavicles and the free floating ribs 11, and 12, are the least likely to be fractured. 0.5 per cent of people have an accessory rib attached to C7 which may cause pressure on the brachial plexus or subclavian artery so leading to parasthesiae or vascular problems in the arms.

Each typical rib has the structures shown in the diagram below.

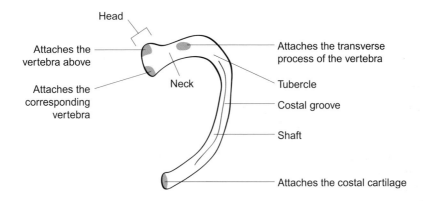

19. Below is a diagram of an intercostal space

    a. Label the three layers of muscles
    b. Label the parietal pleura
    c. For **(a)** indicate the direction of their muscle fibres
    d. Indicate the neurovascular bundle
    e. Indicate the safest place to insert a needle through the intercostal space
    f. Give two examples of why this may need to be done

Posterior 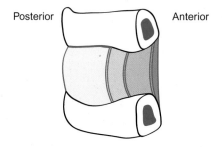 Anterior

EXPLANATION: THE INTERCOSTAL SPACE

Insertion of a needle into an intercostal space is performed when there is fluid in the pleural space, for example in a **pleural effusion**. An **empyema** is where there is pus between the pleura. Another application is if a patient has a **pneumothorax** (air between the pleura), which is treated by inserting a needle in the second intercostal space in the mid-clavicular line **(19f)**. To insert a chest drain if the pneumothorax is not relieved, this is done in the mid-axillary line in the fourth, fifth or sixth intercostal space. Whatever the application it must always be carried out above the rib **(19e)**. This is to avoid hitting the neurovascular bundle. The order of the vein, artery and nerve is easy to remember – just remember VAN.

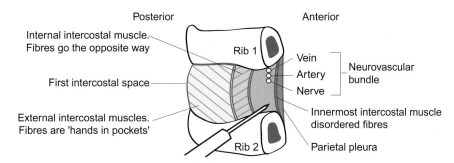

Insertion of a needle must occur at the inferior intercostal margin
(i.e. above the rib) to avoid the neurovascular bundle.
It must also be aimed upwards to avoid hitting the collateral branches.
To remember it think of it as if you need to rest the needle on the rib to steady it

Answers

19. See figure and explanation

20. Consider the anatomy of the lungs

a. The lungs receive both sympathetic and parasympathetic innervation
b. After dividing about 12 times the bronchi are referred to as bronchioles
c. Each bronchopulmonary segment is supplied by several blood vessels
d. Blood vessels, nerves and lymphatics enter the lung at the hilum
e. The bronchial arteries supply all parts of the lungs

21. Regarding the alveoli

a. Alveoli are found in the terminal bronchioles
b. The alveolar capillary membrane is less than 0.4 μm thick
c. There are about 1 million alveoli/lung
d. Surfactant is secreted by type I pneumocytes
e. The total surface area of the alveoli is 40–80 m^2

EXPLANATION: THE LUNGS

The **vagus** nerve (Xth cranial nerve) is **parasympathetic** and has **sensory** afferents, while the **efferent** nerves are responsible for **bronchoconstriction** and **secretomotor** functions. **T2–T4** thoracic ganglia of the sympathetic nervous system cause **bronchodilation**. The trachea bifurcates into the **bronchi** (division 1), which then split into **lobar bronchi** (division 2), **segmental bronchi** (division 3–4), **small bronchi** (division 5–11), **bronchioles** (division 12–16) and finally terminal (division 16) and respiratory (division 17–19) bronchioles. The final dimensions end in alveolar ducts and sacs (division 20–23). Up to division 11, the airway is supported by horseshoe-shaped cartilage structures. **Bronchopulmonary segments** are easily and safely removed surgically as each has its own blood supply and segmental bronchus. They are wedge-shaped and all meet at the hilum and end at the lung surface. Bronchial arteries off the descending aorta supply the bronchial tree down to the terminal bronchioles, after which the pulmonary circulation takes over.

The **respiratory bronchioles** branch off the **terminal bronchioles** and are the first time **alveoli** are found. The alveolar capillary membrane is very thin, less than **0.4 μm**, enabling easy gas diffusion. There are a total of 300 million alveoli, so 150 million/lung. Type II pneumocytes secrete and store surfactant in lamellar inclusion bodies. Type I pneumocytes do not contain any organelles and flatten out to line the internal alveolar surface. The total surface area of the alveoli is enormous at about 40–80m^2, which enables optimal gas exchange to occur. It is this surface area that is affected in conditions such as **emphysema** – see page 41.

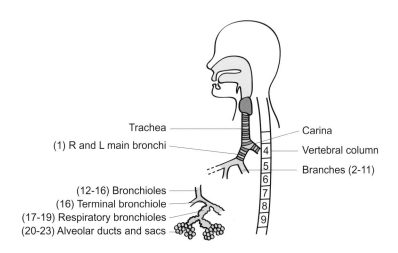

Answers
20. T T F T F
21. F T F F T

22. In the study of the muscles of respiration

    a. Chest expansion during quiet breathing is mainly achieved by contraction of the intercostal muscles

    b. The action of the intercostal muscles is to pull the ribs downwards and inwards

    c. Quiet expiration is solely achieved by elastic recoil of the lungs

    d. The pectoralis major may be involved in forced inspiration

    e. Forced expiration involves the use of expiratory muscles such as the rectus abdominus and the external oblique

23. Consider the diaphragm

    a. The motor nerve supply is from the vagus nerve

    b. It is pierced by the inferior vena cava, the oesophagus and the aorta

    c. The right dome is higher than the left

    d. The central region is muscular and the outer region is tendinous

    e. If paralysed the result is immediate death from asphyxia

EXPLANATION: THE MUSCLES OF RESPIRATION

The intercostal spaces contain three muscles: the **external intercostals**, the **internal intercostals** and an incomplete **innermost layer**. The external intercostal muscle fibres run downwards and forwards (like when you put your hands in your pockets), whereas the internal intercostals fibres run downwards and backwards. All intercostals are innervated by the intercostal nerves running in the neurovascular bundles.

During quiet breathing, ventilation is mainly achieved through contraction of the **diaphragm** which flattens (moving inferiorly) by about 1.5 cm to increase the intrathoracic volume. The intercostals are involved to a lesser extent and expand the rib cage by pulling the ribs upwards and outwards against a fixed first rib. This is often called a **bucket-handle action**. Once expanded, the chest wall and lungs will recoil by themselves so no additional muscles are required for quiet expiration. Forced inspiration requires additional muscle involvement to expand the chest; this is usually achieved by the **scalene** and **sternocleidomastoid muscles**, however in severe respiratory distress if the arms are fixed, for example holding a chair, the **pectoralis major** may help to expand the chest. Forced expiration uses additional abdominal muscles to push the abdominal contents against the diaphragm forcing it upwards.

Answers
22. F F T T T
23. T T T F F

24. Intrapleural pressure

a. Is exerted in the space between the visceral pleura and the parietal pleura
b. Increases during inspiration enabling the lungs to expand and air to enter
c. Is indirectly assessed from the tracheal pressure
d. Becomes more positive towards the base of the lung compared to the apex
e. At the base of the lung is about −0.2 Kpa

25. Regarding lung volumes, use options from the list given to complete the statements

Options

A. Vital capacity
B. Residual volume
C. Tidal volume
D. Functional residual capacity
E. Expired residual volume

1. .... is the volume of air left in the lungs at the end of normal respiration
2. .... is the volume of air left in the lungs at the end of maximal expiration
3. .... is the volume of air that a person could still exhale following normal expiration
4. .... is equivalent to about 5500 mL
5. .... is the volume of air breathed in and out at rest

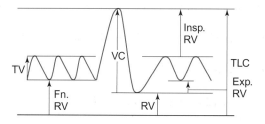

Exp.RV, expiratory reserve volume; Fn.RV, functional residual volume; Insp.RV, inspiratory reserve volume; RV, residual volume; TLC, total lung capacity; TV, tidal volume; VC, vital capacity

EXPLANATION: THE PRESSURES OF BREATHING

The **pleura** is a layer of connective tissue covered by squamous epithelium. The **visceral pleura** lines the surface of the lungs and the **parietal pleura** lines the chest wall. Both join and **become continuous** at the **hilum** but otherwise are in apposition. To prevent friction the surfaces are **lubricated** with a very small amount of **fluid**. The pressure exerted in the space between the pleura is known as the intrapleural pressure. The **intrapleural pressure** varies during breathing. On **inspiration**, as the chest wall expands the intrapleural pressure **falls** – this increases the pressure gradient between the alveoli and the intrapleural space which stretches the lungs and expands the alveoli. The alveolar pressure falls as the alveoli expand, and this forces higher pressured air from the environment into the lung where the pressure is lower. Conversely as the chest wall relaxes in **expiration**, the pressure in the intrapleural space rises and so the alveolar **pressure rises** helping to force air out of the lungs (along with elastic recoil).

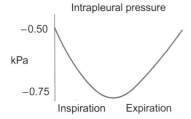

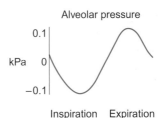

During quiet breathing the intrapleural pressure is always negative but becomes positive on forced expiration enabling the expulsion of air and foreign bodies when coughing. The intrapleural pressure also varies throughout the lung because of gravity. At the apex, the weight of the lower part of the lung hanging down pulls the parietal pleura away from the chest wall, opening up the intrapleural space and reducing the apical intrapleural pressure. Pressure therefore becomes more positive towards the lung bases where it is −0.2 kPa compared to −0.8 kPa at the apex. The intrapleural space is very small, and measuring the pressure directly, for example with a needle, may puncture the lung. It is therefore measured indirectly by the pressure in the oesophagus, which lies adjacent to the pleura (see Fig. opposite).

- **Tidal volume** (TV): the volume of air normally breathed in and out at rest is typically 500 mL.
- **Vital capacity** (VC): the maximum volume of air a person can breathe in and out, typically 5500 mL.
- **Residual volume** (RV): the volume of air still left in the lung following maximal expiration, typically 1800 mL.
- **Expiratory reserve volume** (Exp.RV): the volume of air that can still be exhaled following normal expiration.
- **Inspiratory reserve volume** (Insp.RV): the volume of air that can still be inhaled following normal inspiration.
- **Functional residual volume** (Fn.RV): the volume of air left in the lung following normal expiration, typically 3500 mL.
- **Total lung capacity** (TLC): the maximum total volume of air that can be held in the lungs, typically 7000 mL.

Answers
24. T F F T T
25. 1 – D, 2 – B, 3 – E, 4 – A, 5 – C

26. Regarding compliance

a. Lung compliance is measured as the change in area of the lung caused by a change in inflation pressure

b. The inflating pressure equals the alveolar pressure minus the intrapleural pressure

c. Dynamic lung compliance differs from static lung compliance in that it also takes into account airway resistance

d. Normal lung compliance is 10 L/kPa

e. Lung compliance is increased in diseases that reduce the alveolar tissue

27. Consider surfactant and use the options below to complete the paragraph

Options

A. Type I pneumocyte	B. Alveolus
C. Type II pneumocyte	D. Phospholipids
E. Caesin	F. Solids
G. Proteins	H. Increase
I. Decrease	J. Adults
K. Young children	L. Teenagers
M. Premature babies	N. Carbohydrates
O. Bronchioles	P. Lecithin
Q. Type IV pneumocytes	R. Collapse
S. Fluids	T. Bronchi

Surfactant is produced by 1 cells. It is composed of 2 such as 3 and sphingomyelin. Surfactant lines the 4. Its purpose is to 5 surface tension and 6 compliance. However it also prevents alveolar 7 and the transudation of 8 into the alveoli. A complete lack of surfactant gives rise to respiratory distress syndrome in 9.

EXPLANATION: COMPLIANCE

In order to breathe in the inspiratory muscles must overcome resistance from the lungs (**elastic resistance**). The ability of a material to stretch when a force is applied to it is known as **compliance**. As the lungs are a three-dimensional structure, their compliance is measured as the change in volume of the lung per unit change in inflating pressure. The inflating pressure is equal to the alveolar pressure minus the intrapleural pressure.

When there is no air flowing into the lung, i.e. when the breath is held, the alveolar pressure equals zero. The intrapleural pressure therefore equals the inflating pressure. Intrapleural pressure is measured using an oesophageal balloon while the subject holds their breath in different stages of inflation. The compliance is the gradient of the steepest part of the pressure–volume curve (this is **static compliance**). **Dynamic compliance** is obtained by continuous measurements of the intrapleural pressure and volume during a normal breathing cycle. The pressure–volume loop appears wider as it must take into account airway resistance and so the pressures must change more to force air into the lung. Normal lung compliance is 1.5 L/kPa. In restrictive lung diseases like **pulmonary fibrosis** the lungs become stiff and so compliance is reduced (less elastic). In disease such as **emphysema** where there is a loss of alveolar tissue the lungs stretch more easily and so compliance is increased.

$$\text{Compliance} = \Delta\text{volume}/\Delta\text{pressure}$$

$$\text{Inflating pressure} = \text{alveolar pressure} - \text{intrapleural pressure}$$

Surfactant is secreted by type II alveolar pneumocytes. It is made up of a mixture of phospholipids such as **sphingomyelin** and **lecithin** which line the alveoli to reduce surface tension and increase lung compliance. Surfactant also acts to prevent alveolar collapse; as the alveoli shrink in size, the concentration of surfactant increases. An increased concentration of surfactant **lowers surface tension** and so stabilizes the alveoli **preventing collapse**. Surfactant also acts to prevent the transudation of fluid into the alveoli. A lack of surfactant production in pre-term babies less than 32 weeks leads to **respiratory distress syndrome** at birth with stiff lungs and difficulty breathing. It is prevented by giving the mother steroids before birth.

Answers
26. F T T F T
27. 1 – C, 2 – D, 3 – P, 4 – B, 5 – I, 6 – H, 7 – R, 8 – S, 9 – M

28. Regarding the flow of air in the airways

a. Halving the radius of an airway doubles the resistance
b. The nose and pharynx have the highest resistance of all the airways
c. Stimulation of parasympathetic receptors in bronchial smooth muscle increases airway resistance
d. CO_2 has a bronchoconstrictive effect increasing airway resistance
e. Adrenaline has a bronchoconstrictive effect increasing airway resistance

29. Put the following factors into two lists according to their effect on bronchial smooth muscle

Options

A. Bronchoconstriction
B. Bronchodilation

1. Histamine
2. Adrenaline
3. CO_2
4. SO_2
5. Pulmonary stretch receptor stimulation
6. Sympathetic β_2-adrenergic receptor stimulation

COPD, chronic obstructice pulmonary disease

EXPLANATION: AIRWAY RESISTANCE

Poiseuille described **laminar flow** in smooth parallel tubes as :

$$Flow = \Delta pressure/resistance \text{ (of airways)}$$

Manipulation of this equation gives:

$$Resistance = 8 l\varepsilon/\pi; r^4$$

where:

l = length of smooth straight tubes

ε = viscosity

r = radius

From this we can see that **halving the radius increases the resistance 16 times**. Although each individual bronchiole has a high resistance, because there are thousands of airways in parallel so the total resistance is lower. The larger the airway the more it contributes to the overall resistance. However, outside the lung the airway resistance is dramatically increased with the nose and pharynx having the highest resistance. This is why athletes often breathe through their mouths during exercise.

Airway resistance is increased by **bronchoconstriction**, mainly controlled by parasympathetic receptors in bronchial smooth muscle.

- **Pollutants** (e.g. pollens and SO_2) irritate the airways releasing histamine from mast cells and eosinophils. This leads to mucosal oedema and mucus hypersecretion causing narrowing of the airways.
- **COPD and foreign bodies/tumours** in the airways cause airway narrowing.
- **Stretch receptors** inhibit sympathetic stimulation and induce bronchoconstriction.

Airway resistance is reduced by **bronchodilation**.

- **Sympathetic stimulation** of β_2-adrenergic receptors (e.g. adrenaline, salbutamol) relaxes bronchial smooth muscle.
- **CO_2** has a direct bronchodilatory effect on the smooth muscle.

Answers
28. F T T F F
29. 1 – A, 2 – B, 3 – B, 4 – A, 5 – A, 6 – B

30. Peak expiratory flow rate

a. Is a sensitive test that distinguishes between many ventilatory defects
b. Is the maximum expiratory rate achieved over 10 ms of forced expiration following full inspiration
c. Is normally between 100 and 250 L/min in healthy adults
d. Is increased in diseases such as COPD
e. Shows diurnal variation in the asthmatic patient

31. In spirometry, when considering the FEV_1 and the FVC

a. They can both be calculated from volume versus time spirograms
b. They are both related to the height and weight of the patient
c. An FEV_1:FVC ratio of >70 per cent is indicative of a healthy male subject
d. A normal FEV_1:FVC ratio is found in restrictive lung disease
e. The FEV_1 is increased much more than the FVC in obstructive lung disease

---

COPD, chronic obstructive pulmonary disease; FEV_1, forced expiratory volume in 1 s; FVC, forced vital capacity; PEFR, peak expiratory flow rate

EXPLANATION: PULMONARY LUNG FUNCTION TESTS

The measurement of **PEFR** is a simple, inexpensive test obtained using a peak flow meter. The subject is required to inspire maximally so as to achieve full lung capacity and then sealing their lips around the mouth piece exhale as hard and fast as possible into the meter. The peak flow meter records the **maximum expiratory rate achieved**, which occurs over 10 ms of expiration. The normal PEFR is between 400 and 650 L/min in healthy adults. The PEFR is reduced in many conditions that cause airway obstruction such as **asthma**, **COPD**, **tumours** and also in **respiratory muscle weakness**. It is therefore a fairly non-specific test but can be very useful in the monitoring of asthma where a large variation is seen between values obtained in the early morning compared with those at night. Typically those in the **morning are lower** than those at night. The value recorded is the best of three attempts.

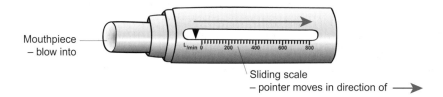

Mouthpiece
– blow into

Sliding scale
– pointer moves in direction of ⟶

Spirometry can be used to measure the **forced expiratory volume in 1 second (FEV$_1$)** and the **forced vital capacity (FVC).** The patient inhales maximally and blows into a tube (similar to the peak flow meter) as fast and hard as possible and until they have completely exhaled. The tube is connected to a pen and paper and produces a trace known as a volume versus time **spirogram** (see below). The values of FEV$_1$ and FVC achieved are dependent on height, age and sex of the patient. The ratio of FEV$_1$ to FVC is typically over 70 per cent in a healthy subject. Spirograms are useful to distinguish between different ventilatory defects. In restrictive lung disease such as **lung fibrosis** the absolute values of FVC and FEV$_1$ are both reduced, however this is proportional and so the FEV$_1$: FVC ratio is actually normal or increased. In obstructive lung disease such as **COPD** and **asthma** the FEV$_1$ is reduced far more than the FVC and so the FEV$_1$: FVC ratio is significantly reduced (see below). In asthmatics this obstruction is often reversible and will improve following bronchodilators, for example salbutamol.

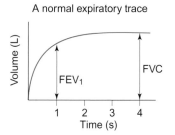

A normal expiratory trace

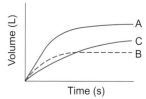

Traces to compare different ventilatory defects

A. a healthy individual
B. a restrictive airway defect
C. an obstructive airway defect

32. Match the flow–volume loops below with the lung defect from the list given

Options

A. Restrictive disease
B. Pressure-dependent obstruction
C. Normal
D. Rigid obstruction
E. Volume-dependent obstruction

1.

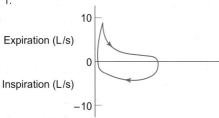

2.

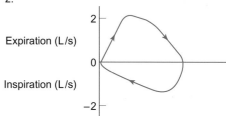

3.

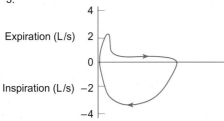

4.

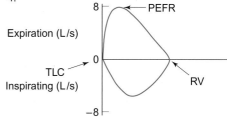

5.

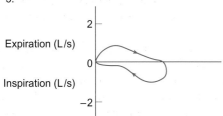

COPD, chronic obstructive pulmonary disease; PEFR, peak expiratory flow rate; RV, residual volume; TLC, total lung capacity

EXPLANATION: FLOW–VOLUME LOOPS

Flow–volume loops measure the maximal flow rate of air in a subject during inspiration and expiration. Their main purpose is to identify obstructive defects in air flow which can be beneficial in the diagnosis of diseases such as COPD, or detecting tumours.

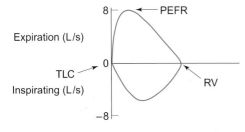

The figure opposite shows a flow–volume loop in a **healthy** person. The highest flow rates occur on initial expiration following maximal inspiration to the **TLC**. This is the **PEFR**. As air is forced out of the lung, so the expiratory flow rate decreases until no more air can be expired. This is known as the **residual volume (RV)**. Inspiration is an active process relying on muscular effort and so the inspiratory flow rate depends on that. It is usually fairly constant throughout.

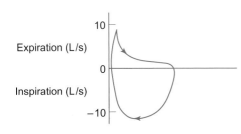

The next figure shows a flow–volume loop in an individual with **chronic obstructive pulmonary disease**. Obstructive disease of smaller airways in the lung significantly reduces the expiratory flow rate. This produces a typical **concave** appearance of forced expiratory flow. Inspiratory flow is relatively unaffected in pressure-dependent obstruction such as emphysema but the patient will actively increase the flow rate to allow more time for expiration. To increase ventilation, these patients also breathe at higher lung volumes.

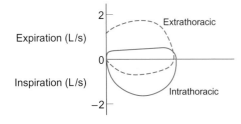

Flow–volume loops for intra- and extrathoracic obstruction are shown in this figure. In **extrathoracic obstruction**, for example in the case of a tracheal tumour, inspiratory flow rate is reduced far more than expiratory. Tracheal resistance prevents expiratory airway narrowing but also increases negative intraluminal pressure so that the trachea is compressed in inspiration. In **intrathoracic large airway obstruction**, the expiratory flow is affected more than the inspiratory flow and a typical expiratory **plateau** is seen.

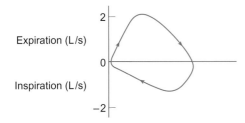

The final figure shows a pressure–volume loop in **restrictive lung defect**, for example palsy. In restrictive diseases the total volume of air inspired and expired is reduced. Low PEFRs are due to this reduced volume of air. The expiratory flow rate does not tail off as much as normal because of increased lung recoil.

Answers

32. 1 – E, 2 – A, 3 – B, 4 – C, 5 – D

33. Minute ventilation ($\dot{V}_E$)

a. Is the total amount of air entering the respiratory tract in 1 minute
b. Is greater than minute alveolar ventilation
c. Falls following an increase in alveolar PCO_2
d. Falls following an increase in alveolar PO_2
e. Rises disproportionately if alveolar PO_2 is decreased and a rise in alveolar PCO_2 occurs

PCO_2, partial pressure of carbon dioxide; PO_2, partial pressure of oxygen; $\dot{V}_A$, minute alvolar ventilation; $\dot{V}_E$, minute ventilation

EXPLANATION: MINUTE ALVEOLAR VENTILATION

Minute alveolar ventilation ($\dot{V}_A$) is the amount of air that reaches the alveoli in 1 minute. Some of the air from **minute ventilation** ($\dot{V}_E$) is held in anatomical dead space so not all of it reaches the alveoli, therefore explaining why $\dot{V}_A$ has to be less than $\dot{V}_E$. $\dot{V}_E$ increases in response to a rise in alveolar P_{CO_2} in an attempt to lower it. However, little response is seen by increasing alveolar P_{O_2}. Decreasing the P_{O_2}, on the other hand, causes the chemoreceptors to be more sensitive to any increase in CO_2 leading to an increase in $\dot{V}_E$.

Answers
33. T T F F T

RESPIRATORY PHYSIOLOGY

RESPIRATORY PHYSIOLOGY

1. Consider the gas laws

a. Dalton's law states that the total pressure of two unreactive gases in a container is the product of their partial pressures

b. The Po_2 of inspired air is less than in ambient air

c. Alveolar Po_2 and arterial blood Po_2 are almost the same

d. O_2 is needed by the electron transport chain to produce ADP

e. CO_2 passes from the mixed venous blood in the lungs out of the blood into the alveolar gas by passive diffusion

2. Given that the atmospheric pressure is normally 760 mmHg (101 kPa) and assuming temperature is 37°C, what is the dry partial pressure of

a. O_2

b. CO_2

c. N_2

3. Why do climbers carry oxygen when climbing high mountains?

4. Regarding diffusion and oxygen carriage

a. O_2 and CO_2 follow Fick's law of diffusion when entering and exiting the lungs

b. The blood–gas interface is 0.3 mm thick

c. The solubility of CO_2 is much greater than that of O_2

d. CO_2 uptake is affected by Hb concentration

e. CO is taken up ten times more readily by Hb than O_2

5. Regarding oxygen transport in a patient breathing air

a. O_2 is readily soluble in blood

b. O_2 is consumed at a rate of about 250 mL/min

c. Normal Pao_2 is about 13.3 KPa

d. It is possible for someone to have a Pao_2 of >20 KPa

e. There is no O_2 left in venous blood

ADP, adenosine diphosphate; ATP, adenosine triphosphate; Hb, haemoglobin; Po_2, partial pressure of oxygen; Pao_2, arterial partial pressure of oxygen

EXPLANATION: GASES

Dalton's law states that in a container, the total pressure is the sum of the partial pressures of the gases, which do not react with one another. There is very little water in dry ambient air, so when inspired it is warmed and humidified. Therefore by the time it reaches the alveoli, the addition of water vapour has effectively reduced the partial pressures of the other gases. There is a permanent balance between the addition of O_2 in alveolar ventilation and its removal by the pulmonary capillary blood leaving the lungs. Therefore alveolar and arterial Po_2 are almost equal in normal lungs! The **electron transport chain** uses O_2 for oxidative metabolism to produce **ATP**. The rate at which this occurs depends on the metabolic demand, not on the availability of O_2 (the amount of O_2 available is usually far in excess of that needed). As there is nearly no CO_2 in inspired air, the CO_2 passes down its concentration gradient by passive diffusion in the alveolar gas.

Dry partial pressure = total atmospheric pressure $\times$ partial pressure of the gas

$760 \times 0.209 = 158.84$ mmHg (21.18 kPa) **(2a)**

$760 \times 0.0003 = 0.228$ mmHg (0.03 kPa) **(2b)**

$760 \times 0.790 = 600.4$ mmHg (80.05kPa) **(2c)**

The partial pressure of O_2 is the same whatever altitiude you are at. It is the total pressure that reduces. So if you consider the top of Everest, which has a total pressure of 252 mmHg (33.6 kPa), the amount of O_2 you will be breathing will be $252 \times 0.209 = 52.668$ mmHg (7.022 kPa), i.e. one-third of normal. If you further consider the effect of water vapour (about 47 mmHg/6.3 kPa at 37°C), this decreases the Po_2 even further to $(252 - 47) \times 0.209 = 42.8$ mmHg (5.7 kPa). This is why it is important to carry oxygen when climbing high mountains **(3)**.

Fick's law states that the rate of diffusion of a gas through the liquid barrier is directly proportional to the surface area available for diffusion, the diffusion coefficient (calculated from the physical and chemical properties of the tissue) and the partial pressure difference at the interface. It is also inversely proportional to the thickness of the barrier (in the case of the blood–gas interface this is 0.3 µm). Although CO_2 is heavier than O_2, it is about **20 times more soluble**, making its speed of diffusion much faster. Oxygen uptake is affected by **Hb concentration**, not CO_2. However, this is only true up to a Po_2 of about 100 mmHg (13.3 kPa) at which pressure the Hb is fully saturated. Haemoglobin's affinity for CO is 240 times greater than for O_2. Therefore the transfer of CO by the lung is **diffusion limited**, whereas O_2 and CO_2 are **perfusion limited** under normal circumstances.

O_2 is very insoluble in blood (0.000225 mL O_2 /ml blood) so must be combined with Hb in order to meet the demands of the body for about 250 mL/min. In an athlete during exercise this demand can get as high as 4 L/min. The normal Pao_2 is 13.3 kPa, although anything above 10.6 kPa is considered normal. A person with a Pao_2 of over 13.3 kPa can only be breathing air with a higher O_2 content than normal. Venous blood is still 75 per cent saturated with O_2 when it returns to the lungs.

Answers
1. F T T F T
2. See equations and explanation
3. See explanation
4. T F T F F
5. F T T F F

6. Regarding haemoglobin

a. Hb contains four protein chains and four haem groups

b. The protein groups bind O_2

c. Each Hb molecule combines with one O_2 molecule

d. Normal Hb concentration is 15 g/dL

e. Generally males have less Hb than females

f. All Hb has the same affinity for O_2

g. More Hb unbound to O_2 than normal causes a patient to appear red

7. Regarding oxygen and haemoglobin. Use the options below to complete the equation

Options

A. O_2 content

B. O_2 capacity

C. Po_2

D. [Hb]

$$O_2 \text{ saturation} = \tfrac{1}{2} \times 100 \text{ per cent}$$

8. Given that [Hb] = 13.5 g/dL and the oxygen content = 18 mL/dL, what is the oxygen saturation?

9. Using the axes drawn below

a. Label the axis for an O_2 dissociation curve and draw the O_2 dissociation curve for adult haemoglobin (HbA)

b. On the graph indicate the Po_2 of normal arterial and venous blood

c. List two factors that shift the O_2 dissociation curve to the right

d. Draw the O_2 dissociation curve for fetal Hb (HbF)

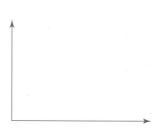

Hb, haemoglobin; [Hb], haemoglobin concentration; HbA, adult haemoglobin; HbF, fetal haemoglobin; Po_2, partial pressure of oxygen

EXPLANATION: HAEMOGLOBIN AND OXYGEN TRANSPORT (i)

The structure of Hb is shown below. The iron in the haem group is responsible for binding O_2, therefore four molecules of O_2 can bind per Hb molecule. Normal [Hb] is around 15 g/dL although it varies enormously. The normal range for females is 12–16 g/dL and for males it is 14–17.7 g/dL. Several different types of Hb exist depending on which protein groups are present. Each has a different affinity for O_2 depending on its function. A patient with an abnormal amount of Hb unbound to O_2 will appear cyanosed (blue) as this is the colour of **deoxyhaemoglobin**. This is in contrast to **carboxyhaemoglobin** (Hb bound to CO), which is a bright cherry red colour.

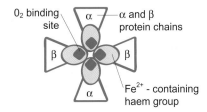

$$O_2 \text{ saturation} = O_2 \text{ content}/ O_2 \text{ capacity} \times 100 \text{ per cent}$$

O_2 content is the total amount of O_2 that is bound to Hb and dissolved in the blood. Each Hb molecule can carry 1.34 mL O_2. Therefore given the [Hb], the **O_2 capacity** can be estimated as $1.34 \times$ [Hb]. So in **(8)** the O_2 saturation is:

$$18/(13.5 \times 1.34) = 100 \text{ per cent}$$

In **normal arterial blood** the O_2 **saturation** is about **100 per cent**. The partial pressure of O_2 determines how saturated the blood Hb is with O_2. This is best demonstrated by the **O_2 dissociation** curve seen below. Saturations must be kept above 90 per cent to ensure adequate O_2 supply to the tissues. The steep part of the curve means that only a small reduction in Po_2 is needed to cause a large drop in saturations. Also it demonstrates how giving only a slightly increased Po_2 can benefit a patient who is desaturating.

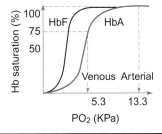

Answers

6. T F F T F F F
7. 1 – A, 2 – B
8. See explanation
9. See explanation and figure

CO binds to Hb **more/less** readily (A) than O_2 as the affinity of Hb for CO is more than **2/20/200** (B) times that of O_2. **1/2/4** (C)of the Hb binding sites can be taken up by CO, and once bound the affinity for O_2 binding to the remaining sites **increases/decreases** (D). This makes the O_2 dissociation curve change shape and shift **left/right** (E). O_2 release into tissues is **increased/reduced** (F)and the patient develops symptoms at saturations over **25/50/75** (G) per cent. Patients with CO poisoning appear **blue/red/white** (H).

2,3-DPG, 2,3-diphosphoglycerate

EXPLANATION: HAEMOGLOBIN AND OXYGEN TRANSPORT (ii)

Arterial blood is usually about 100 per cent saturated with a **Po$_2$ of 13.3 kPa (100 mmHg)**. Venous blood is about 75 per cent saturated with a **Po$_2$ of 5.3 kPa (40 mmHg)**.

Increased temperature, 2,3-diphosphoglycerate (2,3-DPG), CO_2 and decreased pH shift the curve to the right. CO binds to Hb **200** times **more (10A)** readily than O_2 and displaces it from the binding sites. The affinity of Hb for CO is about **240 (10B)** times that of O_2. **Two** of the **four (10C)** binding sites on Hb can be bound by CO, and once bound they **increase (10D)** the affinity of O_2 binding to the remaining two sites. Therefore the shape of the O_2 dissociation curve changes and shifts **left (10E)**. O_2 release into tissues is **reduced (10F)** and patients develop symptoms at saturations of over **50 (10G)** per cent. Symptoms progress through headache, sleepiness, convulsions, coma then death. Patients with CO poisoning have a characteristic **cherry red** colour **(10H)**, they are not cyanosed (blue) as in other hypoxic states.

Answers

10. See explanation

11. Consider the equation below

$$..... + ... \leftrightarrow H_2CO_3 \leftrightarrow ..... + ...$$

    a. Complete the equation
    b. Which enzyme catalyses this reaction and where is it found?
    c. Indicate which of these substances pass through the blood–brain barrier to the CSF

12. Concerning carbon dioxide

    a. More CO_2 is carried in the blood than O_2
    b. CO_2 is mainly transported as bicarbonate
    c. Blood is easily saturated with CO_2
    d. Normal Pa_{CO_2} is 13.3 KPa
    e. Pa_{CO_2} increases with exercise

13. Concerning the transport of carbon dioxide with haemoglobin

    a. CO_2 is transported as carboxyhaemoglobin
    b. The combination of Hb with CO_2 is dependent on an enzyme
    c. Carboaminohaemoglobin is more readily formed with deoxyhaemoglobin than oxyhaemoglobin
    d. Hb is a better buffer when oxygenated than deoxygenated
    e. Oxygenation of Hb leads to the dissociation of CO_2

14. Add to the diagram below to explain

    a. The three ways in which CO_2 is carried in blood
    b. What the 'chloride shift' is and why it is needed
    c. Why RBCs in deoxygenated blood are larger than in oxygenated blood.
    d. Why the rise in H^+ ions does not limit the formation of HCO_3^-

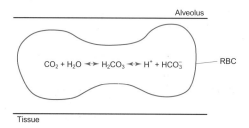

CSF, cerebrospinal fluid; Hb, haemoglobin; HHb, H^+ bound to Hb; Pa_{CO_2}, arterial partial pressure of carbon dioxide; Pa_{O_2}, arterial partial pressure of oxygen; RBC, red blood cell

EXPLANATION: THE TRANSPORT OF CARBON DIOXIDE

$$H_2O + CO_2 \leftrightarrow H_2CO_3 \leftrightarrow H^+ + HCO_3^- \text{ (11a)}$$

Carbonic anhydrase, which is present in RBCs, catalyses this reaction **(11b)**.

Non-ionized molecules can pass through the blood–brain barrier, therefore CO_2 diffuses into the CSF, but the H^+ ions and HCO_3^- are left in the blood **(11c)**.

CO_2 is 20 times more soluble in blood than O_2, so can be transported dissolved in plasma (10 per cent). Also it travels in the form of **HCO_3^- ions** (60 per cent) and as **carbamino compounds** (30 per cent). The most important protein used for the carbamino compounds is **Hb**. Unlike O_2 there is no saturation limit to CO_2 transport as the amount of CO_2 dissolved in the blood and HCO_3^- that can be made is unlimited. Amino groups on proteins for carbamino compounds are limited however. Normal $PaCO_2$ is 5.3 KPa (PaO_2 is 13.3 KPa) and during exercise fluctuates very little despite the increase in production of CO_2 by the tissues. This is due to the body responding with an increase in ventilation to maintain normal levels.

Carbaminohaemoglobin is the product formed when CO_2 binds Hb. This reaction occurs rapidly and without the need for an enzyme. The **Haldane effect** states that 'for any given PCO_2 the amount of CO_2 carried by deoxygenated blood is greater than oxygenated blood'. Added to this is that, compared with **oxyhaemoglobin**, **deoxyhaemoglobin** more readily forms carbamino compounds. It is also a better buffer as it is a weaker acid, so the equation above is shifted to the right. When Hb is oxygenated in the lung, this helps the CO_2 to dissociate and leave the blood, ready to be breathed out.

As CO_2 enters a cell it is converted to HCO_3^- which diffuses out of the cell down its concentration gradient. H^+ ions remain in the cell as they can not pass through the cell membrane. To stay electrically neutral, Cl^- ions enter (this is known as the **chloride shift**). As a result of this and the formation of carbamino groups, there is an increase in the number of molecules within the cell. Therefore the osmolarity increases and water enters the cell, causing it to swell slightly. When the CO_2 is given up to the alveoli, the cell loses its water and shrinks again.

The production of HCO_3^- also means the production of H^+. This would normally limit the further conversion of H_2CO_3. However, Hb is a good buffer when deoxygenated and binds the H^+ within the cell and so allowing the reaction to proceed. This adds to the Haldane effect.

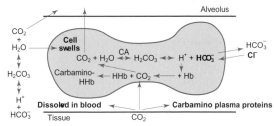

CA = carbonic anhydrase

Answers

11. See explanation
12. T T F F F
13. F F T F T
14. See figure

15. Consider respiratory control

    a. The respiratory centre in the brain is found in the frontal cortex

    b. The respiratory centre is not easily identified on CT or MRI scan of the brain

    c. Opiates depress the respiratory centre

    d. The phrenic nerves are solely responsible for transmitting messages to the muscles of respiration

    e. Respiration is only under central control

16. Concerning the central control of respiration

    a. Transection of the neurons between the medulla and spinal cord results in the inability to breathe

    b. Neurons involved in normal respiration are highly active during expiration

    c. Motor neurons in the pyramidal tracts are responsible for voluntary control of respiration

    d. Higher centres in the brain play an important role in respiration

    e. The glossopharyngeal and vagus nerves send messages back from the lungs to the brainstem

17. Match up the following descriptions with one of the options from the list below. The injuries may be used once, more than once or not at all

Options

    A. Sectioning above the pons

    B. Brainstem injury

    C. Sectioning between the pons and medulla

    D. Stroke

    E. Spinal cord transection

    F. Sectioning below the medulla

    1. Patient has an irregular breathing pattern

    2. Patient is unable to cough

    3. Patient can't breathe when asleep

    4. Patient can't hold their breath

    5. Incompatible with life

CT, computed tomography; MRI, magnetic resonance imaging

EXPLANATION: THE CONTROL OF RESPIRATION (i)

This is probably the hardest topic to understand, especially if your course teaches the nervous system after respiration. It is worth spending a while getting to grips with the basics.

A group of neurons in the reticular substance of the brainstem (the pons and medulla) are known as the **respiratory centre**. They are anatomically not well defined but are responsible for rhythmical discharges and control of the respiratory muscles, resulting in co-ordinated muscle movements. These phasic motor discharges pass via the **phrenic** nerves and also the **intercostal** nerves to the muscles involved in respiration (see page 37). Respiration is one of the few bodily processes where the central control can be overridden to enable voluntary control (i.e. breath holding). Sedatives such as opiates, for example morphine, depress the respiratory centre and, if given in excess, can cause respiratory arrest. Therefore patients prescribed strong opiates should always be written up for the reversal agent, naloxone, in the event they overdose. On the other hand, doxapram and aspirin overdose cause stimulation of the respiratory centre leading to hyperventilation.

Injuries **above** the brainstem, i.e. between the pons and cortex, have **little effect on breathing** as the respiratory centre is unaffected. Those **between the pons and medulla** don't abolish the ability to breathe but **alter the rate and rhythm**. Transection **between the medulla and spinal cord** cuts the whole respiratory centre off from the rest of the body, so **patients are unable to breathe for themselves**. Expiration in normal breathing is passive so the expiratory neurons don't have much work to do and are relatively inactive. As the neurons responsible for voluntary respiration are outside the brainstem, an injury to the brainstem itself may leave the patient able to stimulate breathing themselves but they will also have to think about every breath they take. The major problem here is when the patient sleeps; they need ventilation as they can't breathe for themselves. Higher centres in the brain have an important input in ventilation, for example during excitement and alarm the rate of respiration increases and during sleep and coma it decreases. The **glossopharyngeal** nerves transmit signals from the peripheral chemoreceptors and the **vagi** from lung receptors. These are received and processed by the respiratory centre.

Answers
15. F T T F F
16. T F T T T
17. 1 – C, 2 – D, 3 – B, 4 – D, 5 – F

18. The brain's respiratory centre receives input regarding ventilation from several different sources. Fill in the boxes 1–4 with one of the following

Options

A. Spinal cord

C. Pneumotaxic centre – pons

E. Medullary respiratory centre

B. Cerebral cortex

D. Midbrain

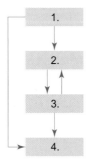

EXPLANATION: THE CONTROL OF RESPIRATION (ii)

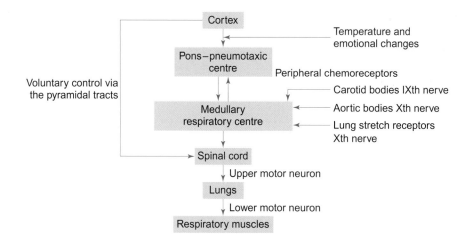

19. Regarding chemoreceptors

a. These monitor venous blood
b. They rely on measuring the P_{O_2} of blood to control the ventilation rate
c. Stimulation causes alteration in the body's metabolic rate
d. Their response to a change in blood gases is very fast
e. Everyone has the same response to a change in blood gases

20. Central chemoreceptors

a. Are located in the pons
b. Are anatomically part of the respiratory centre
c. Are vital for respiration
d. Do not fire during quiet respiration
e. Are stimulated by opiates

21. Peripheral chemoreceptors

a. Receive deoxygenated blood
b. Are found in the descending aorta
c. Are found in the carotid artery
d. Have parasympathetic innervation
e. Are connected to the medulla by their afferent nerves

22. Peripheral chemoreceptors are sensitive to sudden change in

a. Blood flow   **b.** Temperature   **c.** Pa_{CO_2} **d.** Blood pH   **e.** Pa_{O_2}

23. Concerning the carotid bodies

a. These are the most important peripheral chemoreceptors
b. They are made up of one type of cell
c. They are rich in dopamine
d. They respond to hypoxia
e. They have a very fast response time

COPD, chronic obstructive pulmonary disease; Pa_{CO_2}, arterial partial pressure of carbon dioxide; P_{CO_2}, partial pressure of carbon dioxide; Pa_{O_2}, arterial partial pressure of oxygen; P_{O_2}, partial pressure of oxygen

EXPLANATION: THE CONTROL OF RESPIRATION (iii)

Chemoreceptors detect the P_{CO_2}, P_{O_2} and **pH** of arterial blood in order to regulate ventilation; CO_2 is the most important of these. Their role is to keep the ventilatory rate appropriate to the metabolic demands of the body. **Peripheral chemoreceptors** react very **quickly** and their response can change within one cycle of respiration. This is vital to allow our metabolic rate to be so closely connected to our rate of ventilation. **Central chemoreceptors** however are **slower** to react and can take 20 s to detect a change (see page 49). There is massive variation regarding the amount of change in P_{CO_2} needed to stimulate the chemoreceptors, for example some patients with COPD become very insensitive to increases in their $PaCO_2$ which healthy people would otherwise react strongly to (see page 71).

Central chemoreceptors can be found on the ventrolateral side of the **medulla** around the exit point of the IXth and Xth cranial nerves. Although close to the medullary respiratory centre these receptors are anatomically separate and the two are **not neurally connected**. Eighty per cent of the drive for ventilation comes from the central chemoreceptors. They are **always active**, so without them respiration stops. Drugs such as opiates and barbiturates inhibit these receptors so leading to respiratory depression.

The **peripheral chemoreceptors** are situated close to the heart and are amongst the first structures in the body to receive systemic arterial blood. There are two sets of receptors – the aortic and carotid bodies. The **aortic bodies** are found in the ascending aorta and the **carotid bodies** at the bifurcation of the carotid arteries. Their innervation comes from the parasympathetic branches of the IXth (carotid) and Xth (aortic) cranial nerves. The information detected by the receptors is sent straight to the medulla via their afferent axons. Peripheral chemoreceptors monitor the blood flow, temperature, PaO_2, pH and $PaCO_2$. They respond very quickly compared with the central receptors.

Answers

19. F F F T F
20. F F T F F
21. F F T T T
22. T T T T T
23. T F T T T

24. Consider the diagram below

    a. Label the arteries indicated 1–5
    b. Label the positions of the carotid and aortic
    c. Label the nerves indicated 6–8 bodies

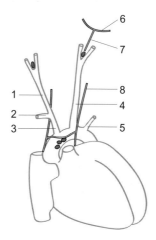

EXPLANATION: THE CONTROL OF RESPIRATION (iv)

In man, the **carotid bodies** are thought to be more important than the aortic. They are made up of two types of cell – **type I (glomus)** and **type II (sustentacular)**. Type 1 cells contain many dense granules containing **dopamine** and are stimulated by **hypoxia**. They have contacts to the carotid sinus nerve (branch of the glossopharyngeal) which is stimulated by neurotransmitter release. Type II cells are thought to be for structural support similar to the glial cells of the nervous system. The blood supply to the receptors is very good, therefore their response time is very fast and can vary within a respiratory cycle.

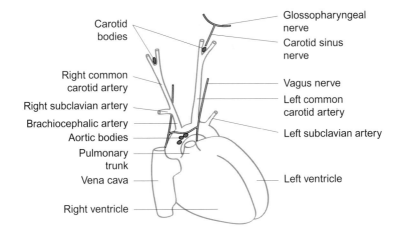

Answers

24. See figure

For the following three questions choose the most appropriate answer from the list below

Options

A. Juxtapulmonary	**B.** Juxtaglomerular	**C.** Stretch
D. Elastic	**E.** Irritant	**F.** Increase
G. Decrease	**H.** Stop	**I.** Constrict
J. Relax		

25. Concerning the receptors in the alveoli and bronchial walls

1. These receptors are known as ....
2. Stimulation of these receptors causes respiration to become quicker and shallower or ....
3. Stimulation causes blood pressure and heart rate to ....
4. Skeletal muscles will .... in response to receptor stimulation

26. Concerning the receptors in the smooth muscle of the bronchi

1. These receptors are known as ....
2. Stimulation causes the length and depth of inspiration to ....
3. Normal breathing causes the rate of firing to ....
4. Exercise causes the rate of firing to ....

27. Concerning the receptors found throughout the respiratory tract between epithelial cells

1. These receptors are known as ....
2. If stimulated in the lower respiratory tract the respiratory rate will ....
3. Stimulation causes bronchial smooth muscle to ....
4. Stimulation causes laryngeal smooth muscle to ....

28. Choose from option A–E which receptors are primarily involved in 1–5

Options

A. Juxtapulmonary	**B.** Irritant	**C.** Stretch
D. Juxtapulmonary **and** stretch	**E.** Irritant **and** stretch	

1. Neonates   2. Asthma   3. Pulmonary embolism   4. Smoke inhalation   5. Exercise

EXPLANATION: RECEPTORS AND REFLEXES INVOLVED IN THE CONTROL OF VENTILATION

Juxtapulmonary ('J') receptors are found close to blood capillaries in alveolar and bronchial walls and respond to **chemical changes** in the lung environment. When stimulated they cause **apnoea** (temporary cessation of breathing) or shallow fast breathing. Also blood pressure and heart rate fall, laryngeal muscles constrict and skeletal muscles relax. They are stimulated in pulmonary oedema, microembolisms and lung diseases causing the release of substances such as histamine, prostaglandins and bradykinin, for example in asthma.

Stretch receptors are found in the smooth muscle of bronchial walls and respond to **inflation** of the lungs. Stimulation leads to **inspiration** becoming **shorter** and **shallower**. During normal respiration they do not fire, but are stimulated during exercise, in neonates, pulmonary embolism and lung diseases such as asthma. These receptors are also involved in pulmonary reflexes, such as the '**Hering–Breuer inspiration**' reflex which occurs following over-inflation of the lungs. Inspiratory muscle activity is reduced and subsequent inspiration is shallower. However, the specific role of this in man is unknown and thought not to be important.

Irritant receptors are found throughout the respiratory tract in between epithelial cells, and respond to **irritation** in the lungs. Stimulation causes coughing in the upper respiratory tract, increased respiration in the lower tract and constriction of the laryngeal and bronchial muscles. These are thought to be involved in the first breaths of neonates. Stimulation occurs following fast, deep inflations and deflations, and irritant substances. Other receptors of note are **pain receptors** which, when stimulated, cause a short episode of apnoea followed by an increased rate of respiration.

Answers
25. 1 – A, 2 – H, 3 – G, 4 – J
26. 1 – C, 2 – G, 3 – H, 4 – F
27. 1 – E, 2 – F, 3 – I, 4 – I
28. 1 – E, 2 – D, 3 – D, 4 – B, 5 – C

29. Regarding the chemical control of ventilation

a. O_2 is the most important factor in ventilatory control
b. The body is very sensitive to small changes in $PaCO_2$
c. $PaCO_2$ levels have no effect on the blood pH
d. Increasing the rate of respiration increases $PaCO_2$
e. Decreasing PaO_2 increases sensitivity to CO_2

30. $PaCO_2$ sensitivity is affected by

a. Level of fitness
b. Morphine
c. COPD
d. Genetics
e. Blood pH

COPD, chronic obstructive pulmonary disease; $PaCO_2$, arterial partial pressure of carbon dioxide; PaO_2, arterial partial pressure of oxygen; PO_2, partial pressure of oxygen

EXPLANATION: CHEMICAL CONTROL OF VENTILATION

PaCO_2 is the main stimulus for the respiratory drive; PaO_2 is less important. Just a small rise in CO_2 causes a large increase in respiratory rate. This is increased even more if the PO_2 is decreased as well as it raises the body's sensitivity to changes in PaCO_2, i.e. it is a synergistic relationship. By using the equation **pH = −log[H$^+$]** and the **Henderson–Hasselbalch equation** it can be seen that by changing the amount of CO_2, the H$^+$ is also altered and therefore the pH. An **increased rate** of **respiration** is used by the body to **get rid of CO_2**, and in a hyperventilating patient too much CO_2 is blown off and their PaCO_2 falls.

Athletes have a reduced sensitivity to rises in PaCO_2. Opiates, such as morphine and diamorphine, cause respiratory depression and so do not react to increases in PaCO_2. Many patients with **COPD** have a **permanently high PaCO_2**, so become desensitized to it. They must rely on their hypoxia as a stimulus to breathe, so always think twice before giving a COPD patient O_2. Like most things, the exact amount the PaCO_2 needs to change by to elicit a response varies between individuals. The body's pH must be kept within strict limits and one way it achieves this is by controlling the PaCO_2, i.e. the rate of respiration.

31. Concerning pH

a. Normal range is 7.3–7.4
b. pH of 6.9 is incompatible with life
c. It is affected by Hb concentration
d. It is affected by Pco_2
e. It is affected by Po_2

32. The following are buffers in the blood

a. Hb
b. HCO_3^-
c. PO_4^{3-}
d. Plasma proteins
e. Iron

33. Consider the following

a. Define pH
b. Define pK_a
c. Given that pKa is 6.1 and the solubility of CO_2 is 0.03, use the normal values for HCO_3^- and $Paco_2$ to calculate the pH

Hb, haemoglobin, Pco_2, partial pressure of carbon dioxide; Po_2, partial pressure of oxygen

EXPLANATION: ACID–BASE BALANCE (i)

The **pH of the blood** must be kept strictly between **7.35 and 7.45** as many of the reactions within the body are pH dependent. A pH of 6.8–7.8 is compatible with life but only for a very short period. Hb concentration is an important factor in pH control as it is a buffer. Changes in CO_2, not O_2, shift the balance of the equation below so more or fewer H^+ ions are released:

$$CO_2 + H_2O \leftrightarrow H_2CO_3 \leftrightarrow H^+ + HCO_3^-$$

A **buffer** is used to keep the pH within strict limits by binding or releasing H^+ ions; **Hb** and **HCO_3^-** are by far the most important buffers in the body, see below for a more detailed explanation. PO_4^{3-} ions have some buffering capacity, as do plasma proteins. Iron is part of Hb but is not a buffer itself.

pH is best defined using the equation:

$$pH = -\log[H^+] \textbf{ (33a)}$$

The pH at which half of the molecules are dissociated is known as the **pK_a** of a buffer **(33b)**. The closer the pK_a is to the pH the better the buffer.

$pH = pK_a + \log([BASE]/[ACID])$

In the blood, [BASE] is $[HCO_3^-]$ and [ACID] is $[CO_2]$ which is $Paco_2 \times CO_2$ solubility. So:

$$6.1 = pH + \log(24 \text{ mmol/L})/(40 \text{ mmHg} \times 0.03 \text{ mmol/L/mmHg})$$

$$pH = 6.1 + 1.3$$

$$= 7.4 \textbf{ (33c)}$$

You can see that if the ratio between HCO_3^- and CO_2 remains around 20, the pH will be unaffected. As these can be controlled by altering renal function (HCO_3^-) and respiration (CO_2) they buffer the blood pH exceptionally well.

Answers
31. F F T T F
32. T T T T F
33. See explanation

34. Below is a Davenport graph. Match 1–8 with A–G from the list given. Each option can be used once, more than once or not at all

A. Normal
B. Metabolic acidosis
C. Metabolic alkalosis
D. Respiratory acidosis
E. Respiratory alkalosis
F. Respiratory compensation
G. Renal compensation

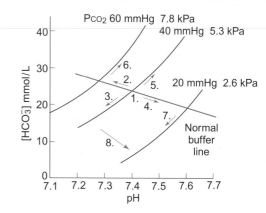

35. Fill in the table with ↑, ↓ or ↔

	pH	Paco$_2$	HCO$_3^-$
Respiratory acidosis			
Metabolic acidosis			
Metabolic acidosis			

EXPLANATION: ACID–BASE BALANCE (ii)

$$CO^2 + H_2O \leftrightarrow H_2CO_3 \leftrightarrow H^+ + HCO_3^-$$

In **respiratory acidosis** (pH↓, $Paco_2$↑, HCO_3^-↑), there is reduced gas exchange in the lungs so $Paco_2$ rises (i.e. in **COPD**, **asthma**). This causes a right shift in the equation and more H^+ is generated and therefore pH falls (acidosis).

In **metabolic acidosis** (pH↓, $Paco_2$↔, HCO_3^-↓), too much H^+ is present (i.e. in **diabetic ketoacidosis** or lactic acidosis). The equation shifts left and $[HCO_3^-]$ falls as well as pH; CO_2 is unaffected.

In **respiratory alkalosis** (pH↑, $Paco_2$↓, HCO_3^-↓), there is increased gas exchange in the lungs so $Paco_2$ falls, e.g. in hysterical **hyperventilation** where too much CO_2 is blown off. The equation shifts left so $[H^+]$ falls and pH rises.

In **metabolic alkalosis** (pH↑, $Paco_2$↑, HCO_3^-↑), H^+ has been lost, for example in **prolonged vomiting** where the stomach acid is lost, or there is too much HCO_3^-, e.g. a child drinking bleach. Loss of H^+ shifts the equation right and so increases the HCO_3^- and raises the pH. Too much HCO_3^- shifts the equation left and lowers the $[H^+]$, increasing the pH; Pco_2 is raised due to respiratory compensation **(35)**.

Renal compensation is the body's attempt to maintain normal pH. When levels of $[H^+]$ are high, the kidneys increase HCO_3^- reabsorption to balance it. Similarly, too little H^+ leads to less HCO_3^- reabsorption.

Respiratory compensation is not very efficient and occurs by changing the ventilation rate and therefore $Paco_2$; H^+ and HCO_3^- are altered as a result. Only partial correction of the problem is possible.

Answers
34. 1 – A, 2 – D, 3 – B, 4 – E, 5 – C, 6 – G, 7 – G, 8 – F
35. See explanation

36. Fit the following into one of the boxes below

A. High altitude
B. Morphine overdose
C. Diuretics
D. Airways disease
E. Hysterical hyperventilation
F. Diarrhoea
G. Vomiting
H. Diabetic ketoacidosis

Respiratory acidosis	Metabolic acidosis
Respiratory alkalosis	Metabolic alkalosis

37. What is meant by base excess?

BE, base excess; COPD, chronic obstructive pulmonary disease; PCO$_2$, partial pressure of carbon dioxide; PO$_2$, partial pressure of oxygen; V̇$_A$, minute alvolar ventilation; V̇$_E$, minute ventilation

EXPLANATION: CLINICAL APPLICATIONS OF ACID–BASE BALANCE

Respiratory acidosis	Metabolic acidosis
Morphine overdose (and any respiratory depressant drugs e.g. barbiturates) (36B) Airways disease, e.g. COPD, severe asthma (36D) Head trauma	Diarrhoea (36F) Diabetic ketoacidosis (36H) Ingestion of acid
Respiratory alkalosis	**Metabolic alkalosis**
Hysterical hyperventilation (36E) High altitude (36A) Pain COPD (hypoxic drive can cause increased ventilation)	Vomiting (36G) Diuretics (36C) Ingestion of alkali K^+ deficiency

The **base excess** is one of the values obtained by analysing an arterial blood gas sample. It is the amount of H^+ or HCO_3^- that needs to be added to make the pH return to normal (37). The normal value is 0 ± 2 mmol/L. When given an arterial blood sample, the BE is useful to work out whether there is metabolic or respiratory acidosis/alkalosis. However, beware, as there can be a mixed picture, so look at the PCO_2 as well. A value over +2 indicates metabolic alkalosis and under −2 indicates metabolic acidosis. This is true unless the PCO_2 is abnormal, in which case there is a mixed disturbance.

Answers

36. See explanation and table
37. See explanation

38. Concerning alveolar ventilation and perfusion

    a. Alveolar ventilation occurs without perfusion when there is physiological shunting
    b. Alveolar perfusion occurs without ventilation when there is a physiological dead space
    c. In normal gas exchange the $\dot{V}_A/\dot{Q}$ is equal to 0.8 L/min
    d. The $\dot{V}_A/\dot{Q}$ ratio is increased when shunting occurs
    e. The $\dot{V}_A/\dot{Q}$ ratio is decreased when a 'dead space effect' occurs

39. Consider the ventilation–perfusion relationship

    a. Alveolar perfusion is increased towards the apices of a normal lung compared to the bases
    b. Physiological arterial shunting increases CO_2 content and lowers the O_2 content
    c. Physiological 'dead space effect' lowers arterial CO_2 content but leaves the O_2 content unchanged
    d. Low arterial O_2 content causes a large fall in the Pao_2
    e. A slightly raised arterial CO_2 causes a large increase in the $Paco_2$

40. In the normal upright lung

    a. The intrapleural pressure is greatest at the bottom
    b. The alveoli are largest at the top
    c. Ventilation is greatest at the bottom
    d. The difference in $\dot{V}_A/\dot{Q}$ between the top and bottom increases with age
    e. Exercise improves perfusion

Pao_2, arterial partial pressure of oxygen; $Paco_2$, arterial partial pressure of carbon dioxide; $\dot{V}_A$, minute alveolar ventilation; $\dot{Q}$, perfusion

EXPLANATION: VENTILATION–PERFUSION RELATIONSHIPS

For effective gas exchange to occur ventilation ($\dot{V}_A$) of the alveoli must match their perfusion ($\dot{Q}$). The effect of a **physiological dead space** occurs when there is ventilation of the alveoli but no perfusion (similar to the dead space that seen in the larynx and trachea). **Physiological shunting** occurs when there is adequate perfusion, but no ventilation of the alveoli. From this it follows that if there is ventilation but decreasing perfusion, i.e. dead space effect, the $\dot{V}_A/\dot{Q}$ is increased. If shunting occurs so the $\dot{V}_A$ is reduced and the perfusion $\dot{Q}$ stays the same, the ratio of $\dot{V}_A/\dot{Q}$ will decrease. In normal gas exchange $\dot{V}_A/\dot{Q}$ is equal to 0.8 L/min.

An increase in physiological shunting will increase the CO_2 content and lower the O_2 content of the blood, as effectively gas exchange cannot occur; CO_2 builds up and O_2 does not diffuse in. An increase in the dead space does not affect the O_2 content of the blood but decreases the CO_2 content due to hyperventilation of other well perfused alveoli elsewhere. Due to the different ways that CO_2 and O_2 are carried in the blood, (see page 59) and their dissociation curves, a low arterial O_2 causes a large fall in PaO_2 but a large rise in CO_2 causes a small increase in $PaCO_2$. In a normal lung, alveolar perfusion is greatest at the lung bases.

In a normal upright lung, the alveoli are largest at the lung apices, however they expand less than at the bases and so ventilation is greatest at the bottom. There is a definite scatter of different $\dot{V}_A/\dot{Q}$ throughout the vertical lung and the difference between apices and bases increases with age.

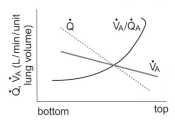

Exercise increases perfusion at the top of the lung and so reduces the difference in $\dot{V}_A/\dot{Q}$ between the top and bottom. Intrapleural pressure is greatest at the lung bases.

41. From the different diseases listed below select the most appropriate causes of

    1. Physiological dead space
    2. Physiological shunting

Options

    A. Haemorrhage
    B. COPD
    C. Emphysema
    D. Pulmonary arteritis
    E. Chronic bronchitis
    F. Asthma
    G. Pulmonary embolism
    H. Lung consolidation
    I. Lung collapse
    J. Severe hypotension

42. Calculate the oxygen and carbon dioxide content of the shunted arterial blood using the values given below

70% of blood passes lungs
and becomes oxygenated

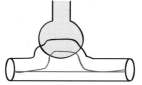

30% of blood is shunted away
and bypasses the lungs

Deoxygenated blood: O_2 content = 18mL/dL; CO_2 content = 50 mL/dL

Oxygenated blood: O_2 content = 24 mL/dL; CO2 content = 45 mL/dL

COPD, chronic obstructive pulmonary disease; $\dot{V}_A$, minute alveolar ventilation; $\dot{Q}$, perfusion

EXPLANATION: DISEASES OF VENTILATION–PERFUSION MISMATCH

In a **physiological dead space** there is ventilation of the alveoli but no perfusion (see previous page) so $\dot{V}_A/\dot{Q} >1$.

A lack of perfusion to the alveoli is caused by a blockage in the alveolar artery or a reduction in blood supply. **Pulmonary embolism** creates a physiological dead space by forming a clot blocking the pulmonary artery preventing any blood flow. In a similar way **pulmonary arteritis** (inflammation of the pulmonary arteries) causes an inflammation in the arterial wall which results in a narrowing of the vessel and a reduction in blood flow. **Haemorrhage** and **severe hypotension** result in a lack of blood flow to the alveoli from either an absolute loss of blood or pooling of the blood elsewhere in the body, for example, peripheries.

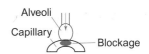

In **physiological shunting** there is a lack of ventilation of the alveoli but adequate perfusion (see above) $\dot{V}_A/\dot{Q} <1$.

A lack of alveolar ventilation is mainly caused by obstructive lung disease that prevents sufficient O_2 reaching the alveoli. Examples include: **COPD, emphysema, bronchitis, asthma, lung consolidation** and **lung collapse**.

The diagram below represents what happens to the O_2 and CO_2 content of alveolar arterial blood when there is a 30 per cent right to left shunt, i.e. 30 per cent of the deoxygenated blood does not contact the alveolar membrane and so does not become oxygenated. Small anatomical right to left shunts occur in healthy people, for example from blood in the coronary veins mixing with blood in the left ventricle, but this amounts to less than 2 per cent of the cardiac output and so has little effect. Right to left shunting becomes much more important in diseases such as extensive lung collapse and consolidation, where blood is shunted away from areas of poor gas exchange and insufficient oxygenation may occur. Congenital right to left shunts are seen in **tetralogy of Fallot** (left to right shunting may be seen in atrial and ventricular septal defects – the blood is reoxygenated).

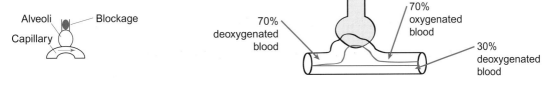

Therefore the total O_2 content of the shunted blood is 70 per cent of the oxygenated O_2 content and 30 per cent of the deoxygenated O_2 content. (see calculation). The same principle can be applied to the CO_2 content.

$$\text{Arterial } O_2 \text{ content} = 70/100 \times 24 + 30/100 \times 18 = 22.2 \text{ mL/dL}$$

$$\text{Arterial } CO_2 \text{ content} = 70/100 \times 45 + 30/100 \times 50 = 46.5 \text{ mL/dL } \textbf{(42)}$$

Answers

41. 1 – A, D, G, J, 2 – B, C, E, F, H, I
42. See calculation

43. Consider physical and physiological defences

a. The nasopharynx is covered in hairs and mucus providing a physical barrier to inhaled particles
b. The nasopharynx protects the lungs from drying out by humidifying and warming the inhaled air
c. Mucociliary transport traps particles in mucus and wafts them via cilia towards the bronchioles
d. Irritant receptors are found in the bronchioles, and cause a sneezing/coughing reflex when stimulated
e. During swallowing the laryngeal muscles relax to open the larynx

44. Mucus

a. Is produced by epithelial cells
b. Is divided into three phases
c. Is gelatinous, consisting of acid and neutral polysaccharides
d. Consists of a gel layer which is impermeable to water
e. May takes approximately 40 minutes to move from the large bronchi to the pharynx

45. Which of the following factors impair the mucociliary transport system?

Options

A. Alcohol
B. Exercise
C. Smoking
D. A low fat diet
E. General anaesthetic
F. Cystic fibrosis
G. α_1-Antitrypsin deficiency
H. Kartagener's syndrome
I. Pollutants
J. Pancreatitis

EXPLANATION: IMMUNOLOGICAL DEFENCE

The lungs have the largest surface area in the body in direct contact with the environment. They are therefore exposed to foreign materials in the air such as dust particles, pollen, bacteria and airborne pollutants. The warm, humid conditions are ideal for bacterial growth and so the lungs are very susceptible to damage. Consequently the respiratory tract has many defence mechanisms to protect against damage and infection.

Firstly, the **nasopharynx** is lined with **hairs** which **filter** inhaled particles, and produces **mucus** to which these particles adhere. These particles are moved towards the **pharynx** via the wafting of **cilia** where they are removed by **swallowing**. This is effective for all particles >10 μm, any smaller than this and particles may get into the trachea and bronchi.

A second mechanism of removal is by **direct expulsion** through a **cough/sneezing** mechanism. **Irritant receptors** typically found in the trachea and larynx are responsible for initiating this reflex (see page 69). The lungs are also protected from drying out by the humidification of inhaled air in the nasopharynx. In addition, protection from aspiration of food contents when eating is mediated by the **closing of the epiglottis** and **constriction of the laryngeal muscles**.

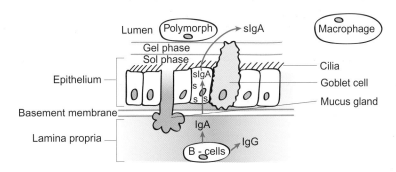

The **respiratory tract** is covered in a gelatinous substance approx 5 μm thick, which is made up of **acid** and **neutral polysaccharides**. It is divided into two phases, the sol and gel phases. The **sol layer** (lower layer) is much more liquid and bathes the cilia of the epithelial cells. The **gel layer** (upper layer) floats on the sol layer and is secreted by **goblet cells** and **mucinous glands**. The undersurface of this layer lies in direct contact with the **epithelial cilia** which move the mucus towards the pharynx by co-ordinated movement. This is known as the **mucociliary transport system** and takes approximately 40 minutes to clear mucus from the large bronchi to the pharynx. **Mucociliary transport** is dramatically **reduced by smoking**, which can increase the risk of infection and exposure to carcinogens. It is also adversely affected by general anaesthetic, pollutants and congenital diseases such as cystic fibrosis (producing abnormal mucus) and Kartagener's syndrome (immotility of the cilia). The result of this is recurrent respiratory infection and ultimately further damage which may lead to bronchiectasis.

Answers
43. T T F F F
44. F F T T T
45. C, E, F, H, I

46. Which of the following statements about the components of mucus are correct?

a. α_1-Antitrypsin inhibits the action of proteases
b. Surfactant protein A is produced in response to viral infection
c. Lysozyme is secreted by granulocytes and has bacteriocidal properties
d. Secretory IgA is the principal immunoglobulin in the airways
e. Defensins are bacteriocidal proteins found in the granules of neutrophils

47. Macrophages

a. Are produced in the spleen
b. Are mainly found in the ciliated areas of the upper respiratory tract
c. Their mechanism of defence is to phagocytose inhaled pathogens
d. Act as inflammatory mediators enhancing the inflammatory response
e. Act as suppressors of inflammation releasing anti-inflammatory cytokines

48. Regarding lymphocytes

a. They are of T-lymphocyte and D-lymphocyte types only
b. They are stored in lymph nodes, tonsils and bronchus-associated lymphoid tissue (BALT)
c. A subtype of T-cells are helper cells that secrete cytokines in response to antigen presentation
d. A subtype of T-cells are cytotoxic and directly kill infected cells once activated
e. A subtype of T-cells produce antibodies

BALT, bronchus-associated lymphoid tissue; Ig, immunoglobulin , IL, interleukin

EXPLANATION: HUMORAL DEFENCE

Mucus contains many soluble factors that help to protect the respiratory tract against infection. These include:

- α_1-**Antitrypsin** which is derived from plasma and inhibits the action of proteases released from **bacteria** and **neutrophils**. A deficiency of α_1-antitrypsin increases the chance of elastin destruction resulting in emphysema
- **Surfactant protein A**, whose main function is in **bacterial infection** where it enhances phagocytosis
- **Lysozyme,** which is secreted into the airways in large amounts by granulocytes. It has **bacteriocidal** and **antifungal** properties but is fairly non-specific
- **Defensins** which also aid in **bacterial infection**. They are bacteriocidal proteins stored in the azurophil granules of neutrophils
- **Secretory IgA** which is the principle **immunoglobulin** in the airway and prevents micro-organisms adhering to the respiratory mucosa
- **Interferon** is a cytokine found in the mucus. It is produced by most cells in response to viral infection and activates lymphocytes.

Macrophages are produced by the bone marrow and reach the lungs via the **bloodstream**. They are mainly found in the alveoli where they form the **main mechanism** of **defence** as there is no mucociliary transport. Macrophages protect against inhaled pathogens and particles by **ingesting** them (**phagocytosis**). Organic material is destroyed by antimicrobial agents and digested, whereas inorganic material is sequestered. Macrophages also clear up excess surfactant protein through the same mechanism. Macrophages both enhance and suppress the inflammatory cascade depending on the severity of infection. In the face of unnecessary immune reactions the macrophages produce anti-inflammatory cytokines such as IL-10. In severe infections they aid neutrophil infiltration of the area secreting chemoattractants. Macrophages are removed by the mucociliary transport system, lymphatics and the bloodstream.

Lymphocytes are also initially produced in the bone marrow in the fetus. During development they migrate out to populate the **thymus, liver, spleen** and **lymph nodes**. In adulthood they are formed in lymphoid tissues such as **tonsils** and **BALT**. There are two types of lymphocytes, the **T-** and **B-cells** and these themselves have subdivisions. The T-lymphocytes can be divided into the CD4+ T-helper cells and the CD8+ cytotoxic T-cells. T-helper cells recognize antigen from bacterial or micro-organisms. Once the antigen is recognized, T-helper cells release cytokines, for example IL-2, -4 and -13. This then activates cytotoxic **T-cells** that **kill** infected cells. **B-lymphocytes** produce **antibodies**, mainly IgA but also some IgG and IgE.

Answers
46. T F T T T
47. F F T T T
48. F T T T F

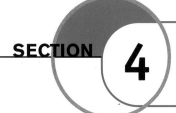

COMMON RESPIRATORY PROBLEMS/DISEASES

1. True or false? The following are risk factors for COPD

    a. A poor diet high in cholesterol   **b.** Smoking
    c. Increasing age   **d.** Being female
    e. Childhood respiratory infections   **f.** α_1-Antitrypsin deficiency
    g. Obesity   **h.** Family history of COPD

2. Two main types of COPD patient exist. They are known as 'blue bloaters' and pink puffers'. They represent two ends of a continuous spectrum. Match the words given to the gaps in the table below to indicate the differences between the two types. The first three sets have been done for you

	Pink puffer (1)	Blue bloater (2)
Physical appearance	Thin	Obese
Respiratory effort	High	Low
O_2 status at rest	Normal	Hypoxic
Typical features		

Options

    A. Barrel chest   **B.** Secondary polycythaemia
    C. Central cyanosis   **D.** Bounding pulse
    E. Cor pulmonale   **F.** Mucus hypersecretion
    G. Hyperventilation   **H.** Hypoxaemia
    I. Dyspnoea   **J.** Oedema

3. Choose the correct type of respiratory failure for each extreme of COPD

Options

    A. Pink puffer COPD   **B.** Blue bloater COPD

    1. Type 1 respiratory failure   **2.** Type 2 respiratory failure

---

COPD, chronic obstructive pulmonary disease; FEV$_1$, forced expiratory volume in 1 s; Paco$_2$, arterial partial pressure of carbon dioxide; Pao$_2$, arterial partial pressure of oxygen; PEFR, peak expiratory flow rate

EXPLANATION: CHRONIC OBSTRUCTIVE PULMONARY DISEASE

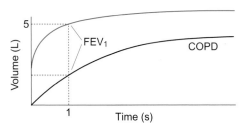

COPD is defined as a **chronic slowly progressive disease** characterized by **airflow obstruction**. This means that there is a reduced PEFR, and a reduced FEV_1, as illustrated in the spirometry traces below.

The single most important risk factor for COPD is **cigarette smoking**, however other associations include increasing age, being male, living in urban areas, low socio-economic status, childhood respiratory infections and airway hypersensitivity. A rare genetic condition α_1-antitrypsin deficiency results in COPD at a younger age.

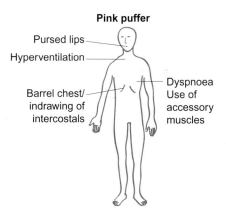

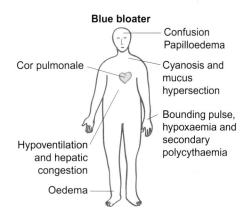

An X-ray of a COPD patient is shown below.

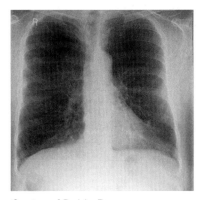

Courtesy of Dr John Rees.

Note increased lung length and flattened diaphragms due to hyperinflation, an aadaptive measure to try and increase oxygenation. There is also a reduction in peripheral pulmonary vasculature compared with easily visible proximal vessels.

In **type 1 respiratory failure**, there is a failure of adequate gas exchange. **PaO_2 is low** (<8 kPa) and **$PaCO_2$ is normal**. Type 2 respiratory failure is due to alveolar hypoventilation; **PaO_2 is low** and the **$PaCO_2$ is high** (>7 kPa).

Answers
1. F T T F T T F F
2. 1 – A, G, I, 2 – B, C, D, E, F, H, J
3. 1 – A, 2 – B

4. Cystic fibrosis

a. Is an autosomal dominant condition
b. Is the most common serious inherited disease in caucasians
c. Has been linked to a gene mutation on the long arm of chromosome 11
d. Is associated with a deletion in the coding region for fibrin at position 508
e. Is a result of a defect in the CFTR protein

5. In cystic fibrosis

a. There is a failure of the Cl^- channels to open
b. There is increased Na^+ reabsorption by epithelial cells
c. There is reduced excretion of Cl^- into the airways
d. There is a reduction in viscosity of airways secretions
e. There is a low Na^+ concentration of sweat typically <60 mmol/L

6. True or false? The following clinical features are typical of cystic fibrosis

a. Recurrent chest infections
b. Steatorrhoea
c. Diabetes mellitus
d. Bronchiectasis
e. Meconium ileus
f. Rectal prolapse
g. Male infertility
h. Deep vein thrombosis
i. Malabsorption
j. Deafness

cAMP, cyclic adenosine monophosphate; CF, cystic fibrosis; CFTR, cystic fibrosis transmembrane conductive regulator; ITP, immunoreactive trypsin test

EXPLANATION: CYSTIC FIBROSIS

Cystic fibrosis (CF) is an **autosomal recessive** condition. It is the most **common serious genetically transmitted disease** in caucasians occurring in 1:2000 live births with a **carrier rate of 1/25**. CF has been linked to a gene mutation found on the long arm of chromosome seven. The commonest type of mutation is a deletion in the coding region for phenylalanine at position 508, which results in a defect in a transmembrane regulator protein. This protein is known as the **CF transmembrane conductance regulator** and makes up part of the Cl^- channels in epithelial cells. A defect in the tertiary structure of the protein prevents opening of the Cl^- channel in response to cAMP.

The failure of these Cl^- channels to open results in reduced excretion of Cl^- into the airway lumen and increased absorption of Na^+ into epithelial cells. Reduced excretion of salt leads to a reduced excretion of water (to maintain an isotonic intracellular fluid) and so **airway secretions become increasing viscous**.

CF is commonly detected by a characteristically high level of NaCl in sweat secretions (>60 mmol/L). Other tests for CF include:

- A faecal elastase test, detecting pancreatic function – levels are low in CF
- A neonatal heel prick test on the sixth day of life (Guthrie test), detects trypsin leaking from the pancreas into the blood – levels are high in CF
- A prenatal immunoreactive trypsin test (ITP) can be carried out in at-risk pregnancies – levels are increased between two to five times in CF.

These tests are only diagnostic in conjunction with some common clinical features of CF; these features are shown in the diagram (right).

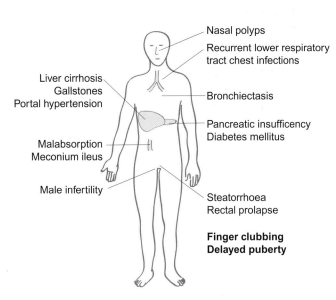

Nasal polyps

Recurrent lower respiratory tract chest infections

Liver cirrhosis
Gallstones
Portal hypertension

Bronchiectasis

Pancreatic insufficiency
Diabetes mellitus

Malabsorption
Meconium ileus

Male infertility

Steatorrhoea
Rectal prolapse

**Finger clubbing
Delayed puberty**

Answers
4. F T F F T
5. T T T F F
6. T T T T T T F T F

7. Which of the following are recognized treatments for cystic fibrosis?

a. Chest physiotherapy and postural drainage
b. Exercise
c. A healthy low-fat diet
d. Antibiotic therapy for chest infections
e. Pancreatic enzyme supplements

8. Other protective therapies for cystic fibrosis include

a. Immunization against measles and influenza
b. Vitamin C supplements
c. Inhalation of recombinant DNAse
d. β_2-Agonist inhalers
e. Psychological and emotional counselling

9. List the features of cystic fibrosis visible on this chest X-ray

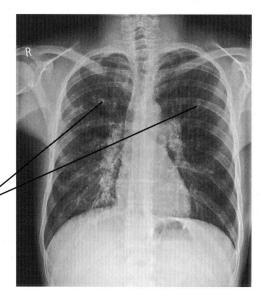

Dilated
proximal bronchi

Courtesy of Dr John Rees

CF, cystic fibrosis

EXPLANATION: TREATMENTS FOR CYSTIC FIBROSIS

The management of CF requires input from many healthcare professionals as a multidisciplinary approach.

Respiratory management: chest physiotherapy using techniques such as **postural drainage** and **positive expiratory pressure masks** to remove secretions is one of the most useful therapies. Exercise also improves lung function. Chest infections should be treated with antibiotics and resistance is common. A third of children have some reversible airways obstruction and may benefit from bronchodilators such as β_2-agonists and steroids.

Nutritional management: pancreatic insufficiency is treated with **oral enteric-coated pancreatic enzyme supplements** given with all meals and snacks. A high-energy diet with protein and fats is essential not only to compensate for **malabsorption** but because the energy requirements of CF sufferers is also 30–40 per cent more than normal. Children are often fed continuously overnight to meet the energy demands. Fat soluble vitamins such as A, D, E and K should routinely be added to the diet.

Immunization: children should receive all the usual childhood immunizations including measles and BCG. In addition they should receive annual injections against viral influenza.

There are also **psychological implications** for the patient and family dealing with a chronic, fatal illness requiring frequent hospital admissions and time away from schooling. Adequate psychological and emotional support is very important. Newer therapies include **recombinant human DNase nebulizers**. These are thought to break up DNA strands found in the viscous airway secretions making them easier to clear. As a last resort once patients are in respiratory failure, heart–lung transplants have been successful, however there is limited availability.

Prognosis: **current median survival is 30 years**, however with improved treatments children today are expected to live until 50.

The x-ray shows evidence of bronchiectasis, which is an abnormal dilatation of the bronchi as a consequence of chronic inflammation. Symptoms include a productive cough of green/yellow purulent sputum or haemoptysis. Radiological changes are linear (tramline) shadows and cystic (ring) shadows. In cystic fibrosis these are often most evident in the upper zones, as seen here.

Other possible findings are spontaneous pneumothorax where part of the lung collapses producing sudden dyspnoea (see page 101) and recurrent infections such as pneumonia or abscess.

Answers

7. T T F T T
8. T F T T T
9. See explanation

10. Asthma

a. Has a prevalence of 40 per cent in the population
b. Is more common in the Far East than in western countries
c. Is characterized by irreversible airflow limitation
d. Intrinsic asthma occurs in childhood
e. Extrinsic asthma is often associated with eczema

11. Cells and molecules involved in the pathogenesis of atopic asthma include

a. Eosinophils
b. Increased number of Th$_2$ lymphocytes
c. IgE
d. IgM
e. Histamine

12. The airway narrowing seen in asthma is due to

a. Bronchial muscle contraction
b. Increased levels of circulating adrenaline
c. Increased mucus production
d. Mucosal inflammation and swelling
e. Structural changes in the tracheal cartilage

13. Characteristic features of asthma include

a. Anaemia
b. Wheeze
c. Nocturnal coughing
d. Upper respiratory tract infections
e. Episodic dyspnoea

Ig, immunoglubulin; Th$_2$, T helper type 2 lymphocytes

EXPLANATION: ASTHMA (i)

Asthma is a disease of **chronic episodic airflow obstruction** which is often **reversible**. It is an **inflammatory condition** characterized by an increased sensitivity of the bronchi to an external stimulus which leads to a rapid narrowing of the airways. Currently, approximately 10 per cent of children and 5 per cent of adults are affected in the UK but the prevalence is rising. Asthma appears to be a disease of western cultures with an increased prevalence in New Zealand and the UK compared with China and Malaysia.

There are two main types of asthma: **intrinsic** and **extrinsic**. Differences between them are listed below:

	Intrinsic asthma	Extrinsic asthma
Pathogenesis	Abnormal autonomic regulation of airways	Abnormal immune reaction (atopic)
Character	Chronic	Intermittent/seasonal variation
Onset	Late	Early
Levels of IgE	Normal	Raised
Family History	None	Present
Response to β_2-agonists	Variable	Improves
Associations	Drug hypersensitivity	Hayfever/eczema

Extrinsic asthma is more common affecting 60 per cent of asthmatics. In addition there is also an occupational asthma which improves on weekends and holidays. Typically workers with plastics and textiles are affected.

The pathogenesis of asthma in response to allergen exposure has two stages. The early phase (1–2 hours) is shown in the diagram below. In the late phase (6 hours later), eosinophil and lymphocyte infiltration of bronchial mucosa occurs. **Eosinophil breakdown** products increase **bronchial inflammation**.

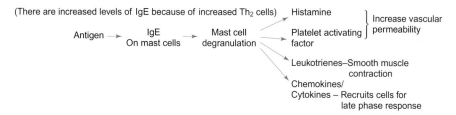

Consequences are bronchial muscle contraction, increased mucus production and mucosal inflammation/ swelling and airway narrowing.

Clinical features are episodic **dyspnoea** (breathlessnes), **wheeze** and **nocturnal coughing**.

Answers
10. F F F F T
11. T T T F T
12. T F T T F
13. F T T F T

14. Trigger factors for asthma attacks include

a. Aspirin
b. Cigarette smoke
c. Exercise
d. Dog hairs
e. Respiratory infections

15. Match the following investigations for chronic asthma with the correct description from the list below

Options

A. Lung function tests
B. Histamine provocation tests
C. Peak flow charts
D. Skin prick tests
E. Chest radiographs

1. .... that demonstrate an improvement in FEV_1 or PEFR of more than 15 per cent following the inhalation of a bronchodilator are diagnostic for asthma
2. .... are useful to assess long-term changes in the severity of asthma and monitor the patient's response to treatment. Recorded measurements show a characteristic dipping in the morning compared to the evening in poorly controlled asthma
3. .... indicate the presence of airway hyperreactivity; seen in all asthmatics
4. .... help to identify extrinsic causes of asthma in an individual
5. .... are not diagnostic for asthma but may rule out other possibilities and identify chest hyperinflation

16. Treatments for chronic asthma

a. Low-dose inhaled steroids are the first-line treatment for mild asthma
b. Long-acting β_2-agonists should only be used if short-acting β_2-agonists are ineffective
c. British Thoracic Society guidelines state that medication should be started at the step most likely to produce initial control
d. A patient with moderate asthma should take regular oral steroid medication
e. Once good control is achieved, no further changes should be made to the medication

---

FEV_1, forced expiratory volume in 1 s; NSAID, non-steroidal anti-inflammatory drug; PEFR, peak expiratory flow rate

EXPLANATION: ASTHMA (ii)

Precipitating factors for asthma are:

- **Allergens:** house dust mite (*Dermatophagoides pteronyssinus*), grass pollen, pet fur/dander
- **Viral infections:** rhinovirus, parainfluenza virus, respiratory syncytial virus
- **Atmospheric pollution:** SO_2, ozone, diesel exhausts, cigarette smoke
- **Occupational sensitizers:** isocyanates, colophony fumes
- **Drugs:** NSAIDs, for example aspirin, ibuprofen, beta-blockers
- **Other factors:** cold air, emotion, exercise.

Reversibility of **airway obstruction** following inhalation of a bronchodilator is **characteristic** of asthma. Lung function tests measuring the FEV_1 with spirometry time versus volume graphs, or PEFR with a peak flow meter detect an improvement of more than 15 per cent following inhalation of a bronchodilator such as salbutamol. Reversibility may not be demonstrated in very severe disease. Peak flow charts are used to record a patient's PEFR throughout the day.

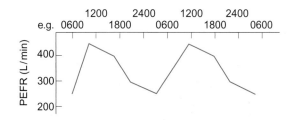

Histamine provocation tests confirm the presence of bronchial hyperreactivity. Patients inhale increasing concentrations of histamine. In asthmatics, this induces a transient episode of airway obstruction measured by a reduced FEV_1. It should be carried out in hospital because of the potential risks of inducing an asthma attack.

Skin prick tests introduce a small amount of a **specific allergen** under the skin with a small scratch. Those that produce a large weal correspond to a precipitating factor.

The British Thoracic Society stepwise guide to the treatment of asthma is shown here. Entry should be at a step likely to produce initial control.

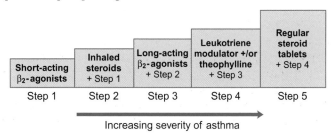

---

17. From the list of options below separate those into features of

> **1.** Severe asthma
> **2.** Life-threatening asthma

Options

> **A.** Bradycardia
> **B.** Respiratory rate >25/min
> **C.** Inability to complete a sentence in one breath
> **D.** Exhaustion
> **E.** PEFR <30 per cent predicted
> **F.** PEFR <50 per cent predicted
> **G.** Tachycardia >110 beats/min
> **H.** A silent chest

18. Appropriate immediate management of an asthma attack would include which of the following medications?

> **a.** O_2
> **b.** Nebulized salmeterol
> **c.** Intravenous hydrocortisone
> **d.** Intravenous aminophylline
> **e.** K^+

PEFR, peak expiratory flow rate

EXPLANATION: ASTHMA (iii)

Signs of asthma severity: in an **acute asthma attack** a patient will often be very **distressed**, **centrally cyanosed**, **tachypnoeic** (breathing rapidly), and using **accessory muscles** to breath, such as raising shoulders. On auscultation there are widespread expiratory wheezes.

Patients with a severe asthma attack:

- Are unable to complete a sentence in one breath
- Have a respiratory rate >25 breaths/min
- Have a PEFR <50 per cent of usual
- Have a pulse rate >110 beats/min.

Patients with a life-threatening asthma attack:

- Have a silent chest because of reduced respiratory effort
- Have bradycardia and hypotension
- Suffer from exhaustion, confusion and coma
- Have a PEFR <30 per cent of usual.

For immediate management of an acute asthma attack:

1. Sit the patient up and give 100 per cent O_2
2. Give 5 mg salbutamol or 10mg terbutaline nebulized with O_2
3. Give 200 mg hydrocortisone intravenously and/or 40–50 mg oral prednisolone
4. Monitor O_2 saturation and peak flows.

If the patient does not improve, nebulized β_2-agonists (salbutamol) should be repeated every 15 minutes and ipatropium may be added to it. Intravenous aminophylline may be started later for refractory patients, however this is not routinely given.

Salbutamol may lead to a reduced K^+ level, however again K^+ is not usually given. Other side-effects include tachycardia, arrhythmias and tremor.

The prevention of asthma attacks requires input from the patient to comply with regular preventative treatment such as short-term β_2-agonists and to avoid external precipitants.

Prognosis: asthma generally improves with age.

Answers

17. 1 – B, C, F, G, 2 – A, D, E, H
18. T F T F F

19. Case study

A 30-year-old postman is brought into the emergency department. He describes that 2 hours ago he experienced a sudden onset of right chest pain while on his morning round. Since then he has been short of breath, with a non-productive cough. The chest pain has improved but worsens when he is asked to breathe in deeply. He has no past medical history or family history, smokes ten cigarettes a day, drinks 15 units of alcohol a week and does moderate exercise. He takes no medication regularly and is normally in good health.

On examination:
- He is a tall thin man who is not cyanosed but slightly pale
- His respiratory rate is 20 breaths/min
- His heart rate is 90 beats/min
- His blood pressure is 124/76 mmHg
- On cardiovascular examination, normal heart sounds are heard
- Respiratory examination reveals that the trachea is not deviated, expansion is reduced on the right, percussion is increased on the right and there are reduced breath sounds on the right.

His X-ray is shown below.

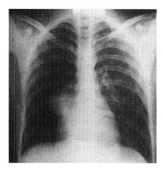

From Lumley, J.S.P., (ed), *Hamilton Bailey's Physical Signs in Clinical Surgery*, 18th edn, Butterworth Heinemann 1997.

    a. What is the diagnosis?
    b. What are the differentials?
    c. Who else is at risk from this condition?
    d. How would you treat him?
    e. What advice would you give him?

COPD, chronic obstructive pulmonary disease; TB, tuberculosis

EXPLANATION: PNEUMOTHORAX

This is a classical history of a **spontaneous pneumothorax**. The patient is typically a tall, thin man (men are affected six times more often than women). During mild exercise the patient develops **pleuritic chest** pain and/or becomes **short of breath** (dyspnoea). If the pneumothorax gets larger (as in this case), the patient's heart rate increases (tachycardia) and he appears pale. If the pneumothorax is small then the patient may not have any symptoms. It occurs as a result of the rupture of a pleural bleb (a congenital defect in alveolar wall connective tissue) which is usually apical. Diagnosis is from a chest X-ray taken in expiration (may also be visible on inspiratory film).

On the X-ray, a black area without lung markings lateral to the lung edge is visible. The attending doctor would use the chest X-ray to differentiate the diagnosis of pneumothorax from pulmonary embolism, pneumonia, pleurisy or musculoskeletal problems.

Other **risk factors** include **asthma** and **COPD** (may present with worsening of their disease so the patient's blood gases must be checked), **infection** (TB, pneumonia), **lung cancer** and fibrosis, iatrogenic complications (insertion of central venous pressure line, pleural aspiration, positive pressure ventilation, artificially ventilated patients), lung abscess (may lead to formation of a bronchopulmonary fistula), cystic fibrosis, connective tissue disorders (Marfan's, Ehlers–Danlos) and trauma.

Treatment depends on the severity of the pneumothorax:

- Small pneumothorax may not need treatment. The patient can be discharged with a repeat X-ray in 7–10 days if there are minimal symptoms, it is the first episode of pneumothorax and there is no pre-existing lung disease
- Moderate pneumothorax (20–50 per cent loss of lung volume – as in this question) should be aspirated (remove up to 2.5 L of air) with a repeat X-ray in 24 hours. If this is successful, the patient can be discharged with another X-ray in 7–10 days and advice to avoid strenuous exercise and air travel and to return if symptoms persist or worsen. If unsuccessful, a chest drain is needed until the lung re-expands. This is sited in the 4th–6th intercostal space mid-axillary line
- Large pneumothorax (>50 per cent lung volume loss) is treated in the same way as moderate pneumothorax
- Tension pneumothorax (positive pressure compromising cardiac output) is a medical emergency and must be treated immediately by inserting a cannula through the 2nd anterior intercostal space in the mid-clavicular line. This may need to be done before an X-ray and followed by chest drain insertion
- Recurrent pneumothorax: surgery is recommended with bilateral pneumothoraces, failure of a chest drain and recurrent pneumothoraces in the same lung (one in five recur in the first year). This involves removing the pleura (pleurectomy) or sticking the visceral and parietal pleura together (pleurodesis) with talc.

Answers

19. See explanation

20. Case study

A 57-year-old ex-dockyard worker presents to his GP with a 6 month history of worsening shortness of breath and non-productive cough with occasional haemoptysis. His wife claims he has lost about 2 stone in weight over this period and has become progressively more unsteady on his feet. He has a past medical history of asthma. There is no family history of note. He takes salbutamol and beclomethasone inhalers. He has smoked 20 cigarettes a day for 30 years and drinks 30 units of alcohol a week. He lives in a flat with his wife and young son.

On examination he looks cachectic and is short of breath at rest. He has clubbing of all fingers with severe tar staining of the right index and middle fingers. He is visibly peripherally and centrally cyanosed with O_2 saturations of 88 per cent. He has marked axillary and cervical lymphadenopathy and a respiratory rate of 24 breaths/min. BP is 120/70 and pulse rate is 75 bpm.

Of note: Chest expansion is reduced on the left. Percussion revealed mid-zone dullness in the left lung and reduced breath sounds in the same region. Neurologically he has a broad based gait. Otherwise all findings are normal.

> **a.** What is the diagnosis?
> **b.** What are the differential diagnoses?
> **c.** What are the causes of clubbing?
> **d.** As a GP what would your initial management of this patient be?
> **e.** Ideally, what investigations would you order?
> **f.** How would you confirm a diagnosis?
> **g.** What treatment options are available?
> **h.** What is the prognosis?

APUD, amine precursor uptake and decarboxylation; BP, blood pressure; COPD, chronic obstructive pulmonary disease; CT, computed tomography; FBC, full blood count; GI, gastrointestinal; GP, General Practitioner; LFT, liver function tests; MRI, magnetic resonance imaging; TB, tuberculosis

EXPLANATION: LUNG CANCER

This case study is suggestive of **lung cancer**. Most importantly are the risks of a heavy smoker (note the tar stains) and dockyard worker (asbestos exposure). Weight loss and the long time scale of the history are also indicative of a malignant process rather than infection. Differential diagnoses include exacerbation of asthma, TB, metastatic deposits from a distant tumour, COPD, sarcoidosis and non-respiratory causes, for example heart failure and anaemia. The nails are one of the first things that are examined in a patient; clubbing is where there is increased curvature of the nail, loss of the angle between the nail and nail bed and increased bogginess of the nail bed. The table below lists the most common causes:

Respiratory	Cardiac	GI
Bronchial carcinoma	Cyanotic heart disease	Crohn's disease
Empyema	Endocarditis	Lymphoma
Lung abscess		Cirrhosis
Fibrosing alveolitis		Coeliac disease
Bronchiectasis		
Mesothelioma		

As a GP this situation would concern you greatly. After a full history and examination, the man would be sent for blood tests (FBC, renal and LFTs and other specific tests for cancer markers or evidence of spread) and an urgent hospital referral for a chest X-ray and to a chest physician. In the hospital a bronchoscopy should be carried out and at the same time washings and biopsy samples can be taken. As the patient also reports unsteadiness and has an unusual gait, this may suggest the possibility of metastases in the brain or non-metastatic cerebellar degeneration associated with carcinoma of the lung. A CT scan (or MRI if possible) of the head as well as the chest should be carried out. These would all confirm a diagnosis.

Lung cancer is responsible for a fifth of all cancers and quarter of all cancer deaths. It is more common in men because of smoking history, but rates in women are catching up. After heart disease and pneumonia it is the third most common cause of death in the UK. Its prognosis and treatment depends on its stage, i.e. what types of cells are involved and where it has spread – lymph nodes, bone, brain, liver and adrenals.

95 per cent of lung cancers are in the bronchi and are histologically divided into **small** (oat) cell (30 per cent) or **non-small** (squamous) cell (40 per cent), adenocarcinoma (10 per cent), large cell (19 per cent) and alveolar (1 per cent). **Small** cell tumours arise from endocrine APUD cells and are highly malignant. They are the only type that responds well to chemotherapy; however the prognosis is still poor, increasing from 3 to 12–18 months with treatment. The best treatment for **non-small** cancers is surgery, however 80 per cent of them are not resectable at the time of presentation. For some of these, radiotherapy can be as beneficial as surgery. The 2 year survival is 50 per cent if the cancer is localised, but only 10 per cent if it has spread.

Answers

20. See explanation

21. Case study

A 34-year-old Chinese unemployed, homeless gentleman is brought into the emergency department. He describes a 4–6 week history of fevers, night sweats and weight loss. He finds that he often becomes quite breathless and has a productive cough that is occasionally tinged with blood. He also describes some pleuritic chest pain on the right (worse on breathing in). He has no significant past medical history but has been hospitalised once the previous year in China for a febrile illness and skin rash affecting his legs. He is currently taking no medication except for a few paracetamol for the pain, and has no known drug allergies. He currently lives on the street with his girlfriend having been kicked out of the local hostel. He smokes 40 cigarettes and drinks 1 bottle of whisky a day. He is also known to inject heroin on occasion.

On examination:

- He is a thin, malnourished gentleman who is hot and clammy to touch
- His temperature is 38.1°C
- He is not peripherally or centrally cyanosed but has a respiratory rate of 24 breaths/min
- His heart rate is 100 beats/min
- His blood pressure is 110/65 mmHg
- Cardiovascularly he is stable with normal heart sounds I + II
- Of note the respiratory examination reveals significant cervical lymphadenopathy and reduced chest expansion on the right. The right apex and lung base have reduced air entry. Dullness to percussion is also noted at the right base.

    a. What is the diagnosis?
    b. What are the differential diagnoses?
    c. What are the main risk factors for this disease?
    d. What is the cause and how would you identify it?
    e. What treatment would you give him?
    f. How would the treatment differ if he had been treated for this condition in the past?
    g. What side effects of treatment must you warn him of?
    h. What public health measures must you implement?

BCG, Bacille Calmette-Guérin; GI, gastrointestinal; TB, tuberculosis

EXPLANATION: TUBERCULOSIS

This case study reflects a classical presentation of TB. Of note this differs from other infective causes because of the long history, the classical night sweats and weight loss. However other potential diagnoses such as pneumonia and possible malignancy must be excluded. **Primary TB** is commonly asymptomatic perhaps with a rash on the front of the leg (**erythema nodosum**). This may just quietly form a calcified lesion in the lung apices or may go on to spread throughout the lungs, **Miliary TB. After primary infection 5 per cent will progress within 2 years and 5 per cent reactivate later.** Quiescent forms of TB are more likely to become reactivated if the patient becomes immunosuppressed with drugs, infection, diabetes. Prophylactic antituberculous drugs may be used in these patients. Pleural effusions may occur in primary disease or in association with more extensive lung involvement. TB can also present at other sites such as the **bones, joints, GI tract, meninges** and **kidneys.**

TB currently actively affects 15–20 million people worldwide and results in 3 million deaths each year. It is less common in developed countries however numbers are now rising substantially. TB often affects the disadvantaged being more common in the malnourished and immunosuppressed, and is commonly associated with HIV.

TB is passed on by the airborne transmission of ***mycobacterium tuberculosis*** between close contacts. ***M. tuberculosis*** is commonly identified from:

- **Sputum** samples with a **Ziehl-Nielsen** or auramine stain for **acid fast bacillus.** This initially gives enough information to treat but culture is also performed to confirm the diagnosis and identify drug resistance. This takes 4–6 weeks
- **TB** can also be identified by a **Mantoux test** – where tuberculin (a purified protein derivied from ***m. tuberculosis***) is injected just under the skin. The area is re-examined 48–72 hours later, an induration of >10mm is positive. This test identifies exposure to TB and will be **positive** in active disease, previously treated disease and those who have had a **BCG** vaccination
- **A Chest X-ray** often exhibits characteristic features of apical cavities formed by a circular ball of immune cells that wall off the infection in the centre. TB lesions often calcify and so are easily identifiable as an opacity on the X-ray
- **Biopsies** of the lung pleura and lymph nodes will confirm the diagnosis but are reserved for situations where identification by culture of sputum or other material is unavailable.

Treatment of simple pulmonary TB can be with **triple therapy** of three drugs. **Rifampicin and isoniazid** are given for 6 months. **Pyrazinamide** is given for the first 2 months. Where there is a stronger possibility of drug resistance **quadruple** therapy including **ethambutol** is used for treatment. This would apply to patients with HIV, those previously treated or with poor treatment compliance, or coming from an area where resistance is high. Multidrug resistant organisms are a particular problem for treatment. Compliance to a long course of treatment when patients are often asymptomatic is a serious problem.

Cont'd overleaf.

Answers

21. See explanation

TUBERCULOSIS: continued from page 105.

Common side effects of anti-tuberculous treatment are:

- **Rifampicin** – stains urine orange/pink; interacts with OCP, warfarin; incr. liver enzymes, hepatitis
- **Isoniazid** – polyneuropathy (reduced by pyridoxine)
- **Pyrazinamide** – gout, joint pain (arthralgia), GI symptoms
- **Ethambutol** – optic retrobulbar neuritis (colour blindness, reduced vision, central blind spot).

All cases of TB must be reported to the local Public Health Authority so that contacts of TB patients can be traced and screened for the infection. Patients are kept in **negative pressure rooms** to avoid spread to other patients in hospital, particularly if there is drug resistance. Masks and gowns are used by those who come into contact with these patients. **Prevention** of TB infection is attempted by the mass immunization programme given to school children. The vaccine is a weakened version of the infection (live attenuated) known as **BCG** which enables an immune response to form against it. In the developing world it is often given to newborn babies.

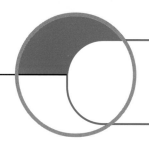

INDEX